The Spa Book

Hairdressing and Beauty Industry Authority Series – related titles

Hairdressing

Mahogany Hairdressing: Steps to Cutting, Colouring and Finishing Hair
Martin Gannon and Richard Thompson

Mahogany Hairdressing: Advanced Looks
Martin Gannon and Richard Thompson

Essensuals, Next generation Toni & Guy: Step by Step

Professional Men's Hairdressing Guy Kremer and Jacki Wadeson

The Art of Dressing Long Hair Guy Kremer and Jacki Wadeson

Patrick Cameron: Dressing Long Hair Patrick Cameron and Jacki Wadeson

Patrick Cameron: Dressing Long Hair Book 2 Patrick Cameron

Bridal Hair Pat Dixon and Jacki Wadeson

Trevor Sorbie: Visions in Hair Kris Sorbie and Jacki Wadeson

The Total Look: The Style Guide for Hair and Make-Up Professionals Ian Mistlin

Art of Hair Colouring David Adams and Jacki Wadeson

Start Hairdressing: The Official Guide to Level 1 Martin Green and Leo Palladino

Hairdressing: The Foundations – The Official Guide to Level 2
Leo Palladino (contribution Jane Farr)

Professional Hairdressing: The Official Guide to Level 3 4e
Martin Green, Lesley Kimber and Leo Palladino

Men's Hairdressing: Traditional and Modern Barbering Maurice Lister

African-Caribbean Hairdressing 2e Sandra Gittens

The World of Hair: A Scientific Companion Dr John Gray

Salon Management Martin Green

Beauty Therapy

Beauty Therapy: The Foundations – The Official Guide to Level 2
Lorraine Nordmann

Professional Beauty Therapy: The Official Guide to Level 3
Lorraine Nordmann, Lorraine Appleyard and Pamela Linforth

Aromatherapy for the Beauty Therapist Valerie Ann Worwood

Indian Head Massage Muriel Burnham-Airey and Adele O'Keefe

The Official Guide to Body Massage Adele O'Keefe

An Holistic Guide to Anatomy and Physiology Tina Parsons

The Encyclopedia of Nails Jacqui Jefford and Anne Swain

Nail Artistry Jacqui Jefford, Sue Marsh and Anne Swain

The Complete Nail Technician Marian Newman

The World of Skin Care: A Scientific Companion Dr John Gray

Safety in the Salon Elaine Almond

A Holistic Guide to Reflexology Tina Parsons

Nutrition: A Practical Approach Suzanne Le Quesne

The Spa Book:
The Official Guide
to Spa Therapy

Jane Crebbin-Bailey
Dr John Harcup
John Harrington

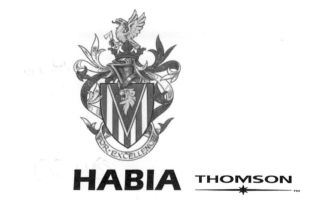

HABIA   THOMSON

Australia • Canada • Mexico • Singapore • Spain • United Kingdom • United States

THOMSON

The Spa Book: The Official Guide to Spa Therapy

Copyright © Jane Crebbin-Bailey, Dr John Harcup, John Harrington 2005

The Thomson logo is a trademark used herein under licence.

For more information, contact Thomson Learning, High Holborn House, 50–51 Bedford Row, London, WC1R 4LR or visit us on the World Wide Web at: http://www.thomsonlearning.co.uk

All rights reserved by Thomson Learning 2005. The text of this publication, or any part thereof, may not be reproduced or transmitted in any form or by any means, electronic or mechanical, including photocopying, recording, storage in an information retrieval system, or otherwise, without prior permission of the publisher.

While the publisher has taken all reasonable care in the preparation of this book, the publisher makes no representation, express or implied, with regard to the accuracy of the information contained in this book and cannot accept any legal responsibility or liability for any errors or omissions from the book or the consequences thereof.

Products and services that are referred to in this book may be either trademarks and/or registered trademarks of their respective owners. The publisher and author/s make no claim to these trademarks.

British Library Cataloguing in Publication Data
A catalogue record for this book is available from the British Library

ISBN 1-86152-917-1

Typeset by TA Tek-Art, Croydon, Surrey

Printed and bound in Croatia by Zrinski d.d.

Contents

5   Spa health and safety   143

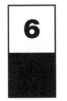

6   The mind–body connection   185

7   The way ahead   195

Appendix A   209

Appendix B, Spa education   217

Foreword

In a busy world we need to make the time to re-energise. For over 5000 years Spa Therapy has been used to relax, revive and restore well being. Over the last few years the Spa Industry has really taken off and it's both exciting and refreshing to recognise this and to include Spa Therapy in the new beauty therapy standards produced by HABIA.

The authors for this brilliant publication, Jane Crebbin-Bailey, John Harrington and Dr John Harcup have woven their individual skills together that set the standard for Spa Therapy.

Jane Crebbin-Bailey, an inspirational educationalist as well as an influential force in the industry lets her articulate and professional manner shine through in her writing. Couple this with John Harrington's immense wealth of industry and international experience working at many of the leading destination and day spas throughout the world and Dr John Harcup's 40 year's experience researching and lecturing in the spa industry and you see the calibre of dedicated professionals.

All the authors bring together their specialist skills and experience to convey their knowledge in the hope that they will inspire you to achieve and practice in this rapidly developing industry.

Alan Goldsbro
Chief Executive Officer
HABIA

Introduction

This book is, we believe, the first attempt to provide a serious comprehensive Spa Therapy textbook for students of spa therapy, practitioners working in spas and spa managers, operators, investors and anyone interested in spas.

Spa therapy, in its myriad manifestations includes beauty, fitness, nutrition, medicine and general well being. It is an area of study in its own right.

Between us we have more than 70 years experience in Spas. The three of us have been involved in the industry from the beginning of, what can be called, the modern spa era; from the late 1970s through the 1990s and into the twenty-first century. It is the lack of published information about spas and spa therapy that prompted us to undertake this task.

In this, *The Official Guide to Spa Therapy*, we have provided a timeline to show the relevance of Spa, in the general evolution of physical and mental health and well being practice. We have ended with a glossary of terms current in the industry in the early twenty-first century. Language is a living thing and the glossary is correct, at the time of publication, but new words and new uses of existing ones are created all the time.

 Fascinating facts are included throughout the text highlighting special areas of interest.

 Tip boxes show the spa practitioner or therapist ways to achieve certain objectives.

Throughout the practical sections of *The Spa Book* we have included step-by-step guides in the use of spa equipment and the application of some spa practises and therapies. However, as this is a fast moving industry and new equipment is being introduced at a phenomenal rate, we have tried to include those that we consider will stand the test of time.

Acknowledgements

We would like to thank Sarah Rawlinson, and her team at The University of Derby, especially Paula Batters and Deborah Flello, whose help and encouragement, since our first encounter at a British Spas Federation meeting in 1999, has driven this book and the development of meaningful spa vocational courses, such as the BSc (hons) degree in International Spa Management, in the UK.

We also acknowledge, with gratitude, the unswerving support and help, through frustrating hard days (and some nights), of our families and especially our partners, James Crebbin-Bailey, Dr Mary Harcup and Shirley Harrington, without which this book would never have been completed.

Our last, but by no means least, thank you is to Thomson Learning whose foresight has given us this opportunity to share our vision and experience – we hope that you, the reader, will find our endeavours informative and rewarding.

Jane Crebbin-Bailey, Dr John Harcup
and John Harrington.
Somerset, June 2004.

Picture acknowledgements

The authors and publishers would like to thank the following for providing pictures for the book:

Aura-Soma Products Limited, South Road, Tetford, Lincolnshire, LN9 6QB, England. Courses on Aura-Soma are available at the Art and Science International Academy of Colour Technologies (AS I ACT), Dev Aura, Little London, Tetford, Lincolnshire, LN9 6AL, England.

Blissworld Ltd, www.blissworld.com

Brenner's Park-Hotel & Spa, www.brenners.com

Center Parcs Ltd, www.centerparcs.co.uk

Chiva-Som International Health Resorts Co., Ltd, 11th Floor, Modern Town Building, 87 Sukhumvit 63, Bangkok 10110, www.chivasom.com

Finders International Ltd, www.findershealth.com

Haslauer GmbH, www.haslauer-gmbh.de

Inchydoney Island Lodge & Spa, Clonakilty, West Cork, www.inchydoneyisland.com

Lesley Munro, Bath & North East Somerset Council

Massor, www.massor.com

Park Hyatt Goa Resort and Spa, http://goa.park.hyatt.com

Phil Pickin, www.photo-grafix.co.uk

Ragdale Hall, Leicestershire, www.ragdalehall.co.uk

Robin Zill, TouchAmerica, Inc. President, Manufacturers of fine spa and massage equipment, www.touchamerica.com

The Rogner Group – Austria, www.rogner.com

SPA of Siam, www.spaofsiam.com

Syntax Design group, www.syntaxuk.com

Stobo Castle, www.stobocastle.co.uk

Thermae Bath Spa, www.thermaebathspa.com

Thermarium GmbH, www.thermarium.com

Topiary arts, www.topiaryarts.com

Tsvia Vorley, Danubius Hotel Gellert

Acknowledgements for cover images

Brenner's Park Hotel and Spa, www.brenners.com

Chiva Som, www.chivasom.com

La Phyto, Tracey Smith, La Phyto UK, www.laphyto.com

Sofitel Central Hua Hin, www.sofitel.com

Thermarium, Gaby Meister, Thermarium GmbH, www.thermarium.com

The Spa, Hilton Hua Hin, Simon Flint, The Spa of Siam, www.spaofsiam.com

Spa time line

5000 BC	Indian (Ayurvedic) medicine. Provides the foundation for a lot of therapies practised in spas today
3100–300 BC	Egyptian civilisation practises water therapy and herbal remedies, similar to those used in spas today
1800–1500 BC	Babylonian culture establishes bathing in rivers and the application of hot and cold 'compresses'
1000 BC	Earliest known writings about Chinese medicine, much of which is still practised
700–200 BC	Greeks introduce cold water bathing, particularly for the Spartan warriors
100 BC	Thailand's (then Siam) tradition of massage and healing dates from the time Buddhism first arrived in Thailand from India
600–300 BC	Persians introduce steam and mud baths
300 BC	Ancient Greeks introduce water treatments to the Roman Empire
200 BC	Hebrews introduce ritual purification by water through immersion in the Dead Sea
31–476 AD	Dynamic period of the Roman Empire
76 AD	Romans build a principal spa in Bath (Aqua Sulis) in Britain
211 AD	Romans discover the thermal spring in Baden-Baden (Aqua Aureliae) in Germany. Emperor Caracalla (211–217 AD) designs the baths, now called Friedrichsbad, which are still in commercial operation in the 21st century. The hot springs come from a depth of 6500 feet and at 151°F are the hottest in Europe
476–1500 AD	The Middle Ages in Europe
800 AD	Ottoman Empire builds Turkish Baths
1200 AD	Knights from Britain on the crusades in Palestine experience Turkish Baths
1326 AD	A curative, iron-bearing spring is discovered at Spa in Belgium – this proves to be the rediscovery of a spring used by the Romans before 100 AD named Sulus Par Aqua, believed to be the derivation of the word Spa

1336 AD	First 'shower' developed in the baths of Bormie in Italy
1449 AD	Bishop of Bath and Wells in Britain proclaims that nude, mixed bathing profanes God's 'holy gift of water'. Bathers made to wear smocks whilst taking the waters in Bath
1500–1550 AD	Renaissance in Europe brings a boost to balneotherapy – as a medical practice
1536–1540 AD	Henry VIII of England closes hot baths and holy wells – due to their implication in the 'superstition and religion of Rome'
1553 AD	First European Spa Directory is printed in Venice, listing more than 200 spas in Europe
1561 AD	*A Book of the Nature and Properties of the Baths of England* is published by William Turner in Britain
1571 AD	Elizabeth I of England popularises public bathing to discourage visitors to Spa in Belgium – which had become popular among the British. She fears a plot to overthrow the Protestant Crown in Britain by the predominantly Catholic population of Spa
1631 AD	Chemical properties of spa water determined by Dr Edward Jordan in Britain
1662–1664 AD	Charles II of England visits spas at Epsom, Tunbridge Wells and Bath which popularises spas ('taking the waters') among the British upper classes
1669 AD	*Natural Bathes*, by Thomas Guiddott, lists the minerals contained in water for the first time
1690 AD	Cold water therapy introduced as a treatment for mental illness
1702 AD	Dr Edward Tyson publishes *History of Cold Bathing*
1723 AD	John Smith's *Curiosities of Common Water* is published in America
1740 AD	Dr Thomas Short determines the effect of temperature on water treatments – made possible by the recent invention of the thermometer
1747 AD	Methodist clergyman, John Wesley, publishes *Primitive Physick or an Easy and Natural Method of Curing most Diseases*
1750 AD	Dr Richard Russell of Brighton publishes *De Tabe Glanduri* in which he claims 'The sea washes away all the evils of mankind', the first recognition of thalassotherapy
1780 AD	George III (the subject of the movie *The Madness of King George*) visits Weymouth on the South Coast of England 'to cure his madness'
1806 AD	Modern massage techniques (now known as Swedish massage) are developed by Swedish physiologist Per Henrick Ling (1776–1839)
1826 AD	John Arnold of Rhode Island opens the first US 'pleasure' resort, a European spa in Saratoga, New York, USA. Saratoga is a Mohawk Indian word for 'the place of the medicine waters of the great spirit'. The spring becomes known as the High Rock Spring because of its dome structure containing mineral

	deposits. Native American Indians believed that the spirit Manitou stirred the water
1829 AD	Vincent Priessnitz (1799–1851) establishes the first modern hydrotherapy spa, with a health package of treatments, involving fresh air, cold water, diet and exercise, in Grafenberg, Germany. This is now Jesenik in the Czech Republic
1842 AD	Drs Wilson and Gully open Grafenburg House in Malvern, England, following the teachings of Vincent Priessnitz
1843 AD	Two 'water cure establishments' open in New York city based on Vincent Priessnitz's principles
1848 AD	30 similar 'institutions' open in nine states on the eastern seaboard of America
1851 AD	The American Hydropathic Institute, said to be the first medical school based on water cure principle, opens in New York
1861 AD	Dr William Winternitz, known as the father of scientific hydrotherapy, opens a clinic and Institute of Hydrotherapy in Vienna, Austria
1870 AD	A Dutch doctor, Johann Mezgner (1839–1909) employs massage in rehabilitation which becomes accepted in medicine in many countries, especially Germany and America
1880 AD	Father Sebastian Kneipp starts practising hydrotherapy for the benefit of the poor in Bad Worishofen, Germany. His treatment centre still operates today
1892 AD	Father Kneipp publishes *My Water Cure*, adding plant therapy and lifestyle changes to the Priessnitz regime
1894 AD	Society of Trained Masseuses formed
1906 AD	Dr John Scheel of New York coins the description 'naturopathy' to describe natural medical cures, including the use of water
1914–1918 AD	War-wounded rehabilitated in UK spas
1917 AD	The British Spas Federation (BSF) formed by 8 spa towns as founder members in the UK
1920 AD	The Institute of Massage and Remedial Exercise established in the UK. This amalgamates with the Society of Trained Masseuses (see 1894 above) receiving a Royal Charter to become The Chartered Society of Massage and Medical Gymnastics. In 1943 the name is changed to The Chartered Society of Physiotherapists
1924 AD	The first facility for remedial exercise in water – The Hubbard Tank – developed by American orthopaedic surgeon Mr L. W. Hubbard – famous for treating the American President, wheelchair-bound polio sufferer, Franklin D. Roosevelt
1925 AD	The naturopath Stanley Leif opens Champneys Cure Resort (as it was known then) in Tring, Hertfordshire, UK
1991 AD	The International Spa Association (ISPA) founded in America
1993 AD	The UK-based Steiner Leisure Group open the first Spa at Sea on board the cruise liner QEII. Leading the way

	for more than 200 Spas at Sea to be built on board cruise ships over the next ten years
1993 AD	The first 'destination spas' in Asia open; these are: • The Oriental, Bangkok, Thailand • The Banyon Tree, Phuket, Thailand • Chiva-Som, Hua Hin, Thailand which signals the start of the boom in spa building throughout Asia
1995 AD	The European Spa Association (ESPA) is founded by The German Spa Association (DBV), The British Spas Federation (BSF) and Le Federation Internationale du Thermalisme et du Climatisme (FITEC) and others
2001 AD	The University of Derby introduce the first degree course in international spa management as a part of The School of Hospitality, Leisure and Tourism
2002 AD	Champneys Health Resort in Tring, Hertfordshire, acquired by the The Purdew Group, which together with Henlow Grange, Springs Health Hydro, Forest Mere Health Resort and Inglewood Health Hydro creates the largest spa group in Europe
2004 AD	The British Spa Federation changes its name to The Spa Business Association to become the inclusive representative body for the Spa industry in the UK and Ireland.

History of spas

Water through the ages

Water has been associated with medicine, magic and religion since the beginning of recorded history. **Balneotherapy**, or medical treatment by bathing and immersion in water, especially in mineral water, is one of the oldest treatments known to man and is the foundation of the modern spa. The writings of many ancient civilisations – Babylonian, Egyptian, Greek, Hebrew, Persian and Chinese – all mention the healing properties of water.

Amongst the ancient civilisations, the Babylonians established baths, the application of hot and cold compresses and bathing in rivers. The water rituals were dedicated to the goddess Ea, who was said to reside in the waters upon which the earth floated. Around 2000 BC, the Babylonian word A-Zu was said to signify a physician and to be derived from the earlier Sumerian A-Su meaning 'one who knows water'. The Hebrews of the Old Testament thought that disease came from demons and was a punishment for sin. This led to ritual purification by water being a feature of the Hebrew religion, subsequently taken up by a number of other religions. Early Indian medicine used water as a treatment for many diseases. Water was personified in Indian religions in the goddess Varuna.

Thus, several early cultures believed that water had both miraculous and spiritual power. Religion and water were closely connected for centuries.

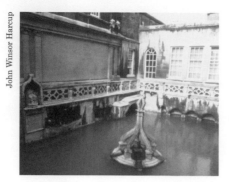

Roman Spa, Bath, Somerset, UK

Greeks and Romans

The attitude to water of the Ancient Greeks was different. By the time of Pericles in the fifth century BC, the Greeks believed that water had the power to heal because of its physical properties.

Hippocrates, the most famous of all the early physicians, following the cult of Asclepios, the god of healing, advised both hot and cold bathing, but warned against extremes of temperature. He advocated cold baths, but only for those accustomed to them. Hippocrates observed that cold water poured over the head induced sleep and relieved pain in the eyes and ears. He was the first to record the rule of opposites: 'cold affusions [pouring of water upon the body] recall the heat'. The Spartans, famed for their fitness, were said to plunge daily into a cold river in order to keep fit.

Galen (129–201 AD), another famous and influential doctor, used baths and affusions of varying temperatures, often alternating hot and cold. His influence on medicine lasted for many centuries.

The Greeks and Romans, in common with other religions, including Judaism, recognised a relationship between personal hygiene and health. However, the Romans took this a stage further and bathing establishments became the centre of their social life. Roman baths included a frigidarium with a cold plunge pool, a tepidarium, which was warmer, and a **caldarium** or hot bath. There were separate facilities for men and women. All these types of bath can be seen in the city of Bath in the UK, which is one of the best preserved original Roman bathhouses in Europe and includes a large, circular cold pool. The water still flows through pipes laid by a Roman plumber in about 110 AD!

From the third century BC, Greek doctors came to Rome and a number, including Soranus (c.98–138), advised water treatment for a wide variety of diseases, such as gout, skin complaints, stomach problems and disorders of the kidneys and urinary tract.

For swelling of the body with water, especially in the legs (called **oedema**), Celsus, a doctor practising in Rome from 14 to 37 AD, prescribed, quite correctly, immersion up to the neck in a cold bath. A semi-circular bath where this could be performed is still to be seen near the Great Bath in the Roman ruins at Bath.

Another Greek physician, Askelepiades, was such an ardent advocate of cold water that he was known as 'the cold water giver' by the historian, Pliny the Elder. The most famous cold water cure was recorded in 23 AD, when Antonius

Musa restored the health of the Emperor Augustus, who was said to be suffering from 'a diseased liver'. As all other treatment had failed, Antonius turned to the Hippocratic principle of opposites and ordered repeated cold baths. Augustus was restored to health and erected a statue of the good doctor next to the god of healing. In his gratitude he also exempted Antonius from taxes!

The Dark Ages

By the eighth century, the Muslim world was developing its own patterns of cleanliness and built Roman-style baths in western Asia. Knights on the Crusades four centuries later were to discover the delights and advantages of warm baths.

It is not known whether the 'sweat houses', or 'stews' as hot baths were called in riverside London, were derived from this Crusader contact with the East. They operated under the authority of the Lord Bishop of Winchester and were manned by barbers, who washed and bled their clientele. Eventually, these places degenerated into brothels, which ironically led to the spread of sexually transmitted diseases such as syphilis.

As the Roman Empire declined, so did the use of baths for hygienic, medical and social reasons. When Christianity swept through England and Wales, pagan wells were transformed, almost overnight, into holy wells, dedicated to saints who had wrought miracles at the site, shed their blood or been martyred near the water source. Other dedications were to 'Our Lady, the Blessed Virgin Mary'. These became places of pilgrimage and veneration. By the Middle Ages there were over 30 major sites of pilgrimage in the UK; the most famous was St Winifred's Well at Holywell in Clwyd, North Wales. Today, St Winifred's possesses the only well building where immersion is possible to have survived the Reformation. In addition, there were numerous minor sites known locally where drinking the water or bathing in it was said to be efficacious for a host of medical conditions.

The Middle Ages

Throughout the Middle Ages (1000–1400), only the medical school at Salerno, Italy, retained the Hippocratic traditions and the use of cold water, although some Arab doctors also championed cold baths at this time. However, it was during this period that warm springs were developed in Central Europe, including those in Buda (later Budapest). In Bohemia, at Teplice, the waters became renowned for

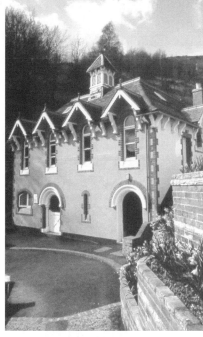

John Winsor Harcup

Holywell, Malvern, UK

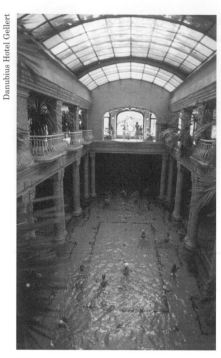

Danubius Hotel Gellert

The Gellert Spa, Budapest, Hungary

healing the wounds of soldiers. But, the most famous spa in this area was Carlsbad (now known as Karlovy Vary in the Czech Republic), 'found' by Emperor Charles IV whilst out hunting in 1347. It became so popular that by 1351 a Cure Tax was levied!

Different methods of administering water began to be devised.

The douche (from *docciare* – to pour by drops), or shower as we know it today, was first used by Pieto Tussignano at the baths of Bormio in Italy around 1336. Paracelsus (1493–1541), a chemist famous for breaking with the traditions of Greek medicine, which were still strongly adhered to up to this time, continued to advocate cold as well as hot bathing for certain diseases.

Hot baths and mixed bathing

By the fourteenth century, hot springs in England had fallen into disrepute, because of nude, mixed bathing, which contributed to the spread of diseases such as syphilis, leprosy and plague, via blood-letting (venesection) and enemas (clysters), which were often administered whilst the patient was actually in the water.

These factors were compounded by the immoral behaviour exhibited by the bathers. In 1449, the Bishop of Bath and Wells was of the opinion that nude, mixed bathing profaned God's holy gift of water. As a result, bathers were made to wear smocks or shifts, whilst taking the waters at Bath. In England, these views contributed to the closure of hot baths or their strict regulation by Henry VIII – a situation that continued for almost 150 years. As late as the seventeenth century, Samuel Pepys, the famous diarist, remarked about Bath: 'Methinks it cannot be clean to go so many bodies in the same water'. These factors and political problems led to the encouragement of cold bathing.

The effect of the Reformation

The Reformation under Henry VIII also closed most of the holy wells, as worship was seen to be steeped in the superstition and religion of Rome. However, pilgrimages to and gatherings at healing wells were long-established customs and were difficult to stop. By the time of Elizabeth I this addiction to visiting healing wells became a political problem – all because of a town named Spa in Belgium, which became famous for a curative, iron-bearing spring, discovered in 1326, appropriately, by an iron-master named

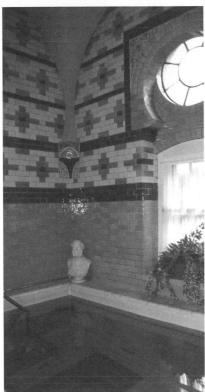

Turkish Baths, Harrogate, UK

Collin Le Loupe, who claimed he had been healed by the water.

The derivation of the word spa is uncertain. Some writers think that the word is derived from the Walloon term 'espa' meaning fountain. The name of the town is believed by others to derive from Roman times, when its healing powers became apparent. The Romans then named the place 'sanus per aqua' (health through water) or SPA. According to Ralph Jackson in his monograph, *Waters and Spas in the Classical World*, the Romans called their major spas 'aquae', of which 100 are known. However, the *Oxford English Dictionary on Historical Principles* puts usage of the word spa much later – from 1626 it meant a medicinal well and only in 1777 did it refer to a place or resort with a mineral spring.

Spa, in Belgium, became the focus for English Catholic dissidents, meeting with other Catholics from different parts of Europe, under the pretence of 'taking the waters'. The government in England feared that plots to overthrow the English Protestant monarchy could be hatched there. In order to limit the numbers travelling, an Act of Parliament in 1571 decreed that licences were to be issued for all visits to Spa. Another answer to this threat was to popularise public bathing, hitherto forbidden in England, whilst actively discouraging excursions abroad to Spa. Active steps were taken to promote new medicinal wells not tainted by superstition or the old Catholic religion. The Privy Council encouraged bathing at several sites in England – Bath in the west, Buxton and Harrogate in the north and a centrally-situated spring at Kings Newnham in Warwickshire, now forgotten.

In the sixteenth century, the Renaissance transformed medicine and encouraged a resurgence of interest in balneology. 'Taking the waters' was suddenly regarded as a medical discipline for the physician, as Andrea Bacci argued in his *De Thermis,* published in Venice in 1571. Other books played their part in promoting these healing centres. The largest, an early spa directory, was *De Balneis* by Thomasso Guinta, printed in Venice in 1553. This listed over 200 springs in Europe, including those of Germany, Italy and Switzerland where the most famous were the warm sulphurous baths of Baden.

Italy also tried to develop its spas during the Renaissance. For example, the famous sulphurous springs of Abano, the Paduan baths with their mud, Lucca and Caldiero.

France was slow to catch up with the rise of balneology; Forges in Normandy did not develop until the seventeenth century together with Vichy and Plombieres. A century later, the sweating chambers and hot sulphurous baths of Aix-la-Chapelle lured the spa goer, but the hot springs of Aix-les-Bains, whose origins go back to Roman times as Aquae Allobrogum, did not have their heyday until the 1890s.

The first publication to encourage the rise of 'the English Spaw', as it was called, was William Turner's *A Book of the Natures and Properties of the Baths of England* written in 1562. This compared the neglected English bathing places with those of Germany and Italy. Turner suggested a walk before having a cold bath for an hour and noted, amongst other things, that it was 'good for all bones . . . and all kinds of itching'.

The impact of science

Minerals in the water

With advances in chemical analysis, doctors turned their attention to the minerals dissolved in water. These 'chymical doctors' as they were called, probed the mystique surrounding the healing qualities of various waters anchoring them firmly to their mineral content.

The earliest work extolling the curative properties of mineral waters was William Turner's book, mentioned above. Discussion of the chemical content of spa waters had to wait until a physician at Bath, Dr Edward Jorden, published his findings in 1631. His work, *Natural Bathes*, was revived and republished by Thomas Guidott in 1669, together with a list of minerals and their qualities. The table described minerals such as stones, earths, concrete juices, metals, spirits and bitumen (a group of inflammable hydrocarbons such as naphtha, petroleum and asphalt). The 'concrete juices' were said to be the tinctures and spirits extracted from the minerals that gave the water its distinctive taste, noted by another as 'salty, nitrous, aluminous, vitroline, sulphurous and bituminous'. As the taste varied and changed on transportation, this led to the idea that it was best to drink the water at its source.

Jorden had also written about the secondary qualities of water – 'astringent, opening, penetrating, mollifying (softening) and cleansing'. He used these properties to pinpoint their uses in the medicine of the day, for example mollifying waters for hard and scirrhous (slow growing, fibrous and malignant) tumours; cleansing waters for internal ulcers; and astringent waters for every type of flux (the abnormal flow of blood or excrement from the bowels and other organs). His main claim was that English spas were as good as the popular foreign ones. Jorden believed that the minerals came from seawater percolating through rock fissures, despite the fact that most of the springs flowed high above sea level. The presence of salt in mineral waters supported the advocates of the seawater origin theory.

One problem, however, was the small quantities of minerals in these waters. Doctors therefore advocated drinking upwards of three pints a day, gradually increasing to eight and a half and then decreasing to the original level over a period of 20 days. Dr William Simpson, son of a brewer, was another of this new breed of doctor. He believed that disease was due to faulty chemical reactions resulting from incorrect fermentation during digestion. Minerals were thought by Simpson to normalise these faulty fermentations.

The minerals commonly found in water by Jorden included salt, alum and six metals – iron, gold, silver, copper, tin and lead. There were frequent debates amongst the doctors as to the exact minerals and salts in a particular water, especially at Scarborough Spa.

Madness and water

In the late seventeenth century the governors of the Bethlem Hospital for the Insane, one of the five great London hospitals of that century, introduced cold bathing for the treatment of mental illness. This regime continued for more than 100 years. At least one doctor is recorded as saying that it was 'much for the benefit of the patients'. Water treatment for mental illness continued to be used sporadically in mental hospitals right up to the twentieth century.

Doctors and cold bathing

In the 1680s Dr Edward Tyson, a physician and an anatomist, used cold baths as a first line treatment. Tyson was consulted by Sir John Floyer, who devised a watch in order to count the pulse, and wrote 'about curing Madness by Cold Baths' in his *History of Cold Bathing*, published in 1702. It was sub-titled as 'proving that the best cures done by cold baths are lately observed to arise from the temperate use of hot baths first'. Floyer stressed the need to acclimatise first to cold water. His first attempt at advocating this was *An Essay to prove Cold Bathing both safe and Useful*, wherein he observed that cold water stimulated the circulation, and promoted sleep.

Floyer appears to have been the first to note that cold water was better in this respect than opiates and discussed its use in 'narcotick poysons [sic] and sleepy diseases'. It is interesting to note that Floyer was also the first to recommend today's emergency treatment for burns and scalds with the instruction – 'immediately plunge the part into cold water'.

Floyer's rules for bath time were 'not to stay in above two or three minutes . . . to go in and out immediately on first bathing after immersion of the whole body' and, preferably, 'before dinner, after fasting or in the afternoon between four and five o'clock'. As for the temperature – that was to be 'as the patient can easily bear it'. The first named patient to be treated by cold water baths in Britain was a Mrs Bates of Ashby de la Zouch, who was complaining of a consumptive (due to tuberculosis) cough and 20 years of 'rheumatick pains'. In 1699, Sir John sent her to Willowbridge spring for 'water up to the neck' every day for a month. He also used his method to cure asthma, 'hysterical fits', though not epileptic ones, mania, melancholy and vertigo, noting that always during immersion 'the pulse becomes slow, small, rare and languid'. He observed that the slowing of the pulse in cold water was proportional to the temperature.

Floyer's ally in promoting cold water treatment was a Dr Joseph Browne who also advised acclimatisation – 'wash first in warm water in May, then every morning in cooler 'till the body can bear the sense of cold water'. He believed that in this way he could cure 'consumption [tuberculosis], dropsie [swelling of the body due to fluid retention as in heart failure], noises in the ears [tinnitus], rumbling wind in the gut and strange imaginings', amongst many other conditions. He concluded 'the muscles of the heart become stronger by cold bathing'. His colleagues did not believe him and opposed his ideas, even hinting that harm would come from his procedures.

Browne countered their criticisms 'against Plain Experience and Demonstrations to the contrary', by citing the custom of the working population of washing their linen shirts and smocks and then getting dressed in them whilst cold and wet, without coming to any harm.

Royal patronage popularises spas

In post-Restoration England the King and court made spas popular again. Charles II was the first royal champion of medicinal waters. Whilst in exile, he had visited the town of Spa in 1645. He returned to England in 1660 and travelled to Epsom in 1662 and 1664 and Tunbridge Wells and then Bath in 1663. These were at the time, with the exception of Bath, drinking spas. By the end of the seventeenth century, cold bathing had developed and spread across the country. Several became famous in London – one at Long Acre was frequented by Queen Anne and another, the Clerkenwell Cold Bath, erected in 1697, was noted for curing rheumatism.

The King and court established a tour of spas, including Bath, Epsom and Tunbridge Wells during the summer. By this time, doctors had realised the advantages of encouraging their patients to 'take the waters' at their source under the personal supervision of a resident physician. Each spa water was said to have its own unique properties and special healing powers for certain illnesses.

About this time, a certain Benjamin Allen was advising those seeking health to 'quicken the spirits by exercise, riding, cold baths and business', thus heralding a new dimension in aspects of the cure by emphasising the importance of exercising both mind and body – as practised in the modern spa today.

The effect of temperature

The invention of the thermometer, probably by Galileo in 1595, made it possible to determine the temperature of the water. The thermometer was refined by several people including Sanctorious, the Duke Ferdinand of Tuscany and, in 1700, by Sir Isaac Newton. With further development and calibration of the thermometer by Daniel Fahrenheit, the temperature of the bath water became an important factor in treatments.

It was Dr Thomas Short who was the first to argue, in 1740, that it was necessary to know the temperature of the bath in order to determine the time that the bathers should stay in it. He postulated that the temperature 'helps the healing properties'. Short observed that 'the inhabitants of cold mountainous areas, can bear a colder bath' whilst 'older persons, females and children bore temperatures of 28–30 degrees'. He preferred seawater to that of rivers, certain that 'in old obstinate pains, the coldest baths will perform a cure more effectually and expeditiously than the milder'.

Non-medical advocates of water

One of the many to recommend cold bathing who were not physicians was the well-known Methodist clergyman,

John Wesley (1703–91). He wrote *Primitive Physick or an easy and natural method of curing most diseases* in 1747. This book, more than any other at the time, made cold bathing fashionable. It ran to at least 30 editions over the next 100 years. He asserted that cold bathing 'prevents abundance of diseases . . . and prevents the danger of catching cold', an observation that scientists are confirming today.

At the end of his book he appended a list of 65 conditions, in adults as well as children, ranging from asthma to tetanus and vertigo, which were 'frequently cured by cold bathing'.

The 'discovery' of seawater

In his *Treaty of Medicine*, Hippocrates extolled the sea's benefits, as did Euripides, Plato and Aristotle. The Ancients, Pliny and Bourzes also observed the oiliness of seawater. A well-known proverb used by the Ancients was 'do not throw seawater on to the fire', on account of its oiliness. The notion of the sea as a healing force pre-dates any hard science. 'The sun cure and the ocean cure impose themselves over the majority of maladies and utmost in the afflictions of women,' Herodotus wrote in the fifth century BC. For almost 2000 years after the Greeks the beneficial properties of the sea were forgotten. The next stage in the modern spa story started when doctors began to realise that the British Isles were surrounded by a therapeutic cold bath.

It was in fact an Englishman, Dr Richard Russell of Brighton, who championed the cult of sea bathing in his book, *De Tabe Glandulari*, written in 1750 and translated into English three years later. Russell wrote: 'The sea is a kind of common defence against the corruption and putrefaction of bodies' (*A Dissertation on the use of Sea Water for the glands and tumours*, London 1752). He referred to the Ancients, who drank seawater, and the Greeks, who used seawater pools to bathe in whilst listening to music.

Russell wrote about the four principal qualities of seawater:

1. *Saltiness* – different densities of salt in various seas – for example the Atlantic, Mediterranean, Dead Sea and Red Sea.

2. *Bitterness* – due to the presence of sulphur and mixes of hydrocarbons.

Fascinating Fact

The further that man moves away from the sea, the more he has to adapt to the environment. You have to live and not just survive! (Richard Russell, 1752)

3. *Nitrosity* – due to the presence of nitrogen.

4. *Oiliness* – not found in spring water but this quality does appear in seawater.

Spas such as Scarborough and Brighton, both of which jostled for the title 'Queen of the English Watering Places', and Blackpool all emerged to demand the attention of the visitor, together with many small and now forgotten coastal watering places. When George III visited Weymouth in 1780, his physicians encouraged him to plunge into the English Channel to cure his madness, thus endorsing the new fashion in bathing 'By Appointment'.

Thalassotherapy

The word **thalassotherapy**, originating from the Greek 'Thalassa' meaning sea, was introduced by Dr De la Bonardhiére in 1867. We all know that we feel better beside the sea. The curative effects of seawater have been recognised for a very long time. The basic principle of thalassotherapy is that repeated exposure to sea air and repeated immersions in warm seawater, mud, clay, protein-rich algae and micro-organisms, such as plankton or sand, help restore the body's natural chemical balance. During immersion in warm seawater, minerals pass through the outer layers of the skin, are absorbed and stored in the subcutaneous (lower) layers, to be released later into the body's system, in a process similar to charging a battery.

In France the benefits of spending time at a thalassotherapy centre are said to be considerable. Many of the treatments practised there are based on the baths and bathing of classical antiquity and philosophies that have emanated from the Orient.

Dr John Latham founded the first marine hospital in Margate (The Royal Sea-Bathing Infirmary) on the east coast of England in 1791. However, it was left to others to develop and exploit this idea.

In 1899 Dr Louis Bagot discovered that when weak arthritic or rheumatic joints were bathed in heated seawater they became mobile again. He had been interested in **climatotherapy** from a young age following a holiday in Somalia. In 1887 he lived in St-Pol de Léon, in Brittany, France, where he studied the area and the climate.

In correspondence with René Quinton (1866–1925), Bagot decided to bring together the sea, rich in minerals, and the **tonicité** of the climate. He pioneered treatments

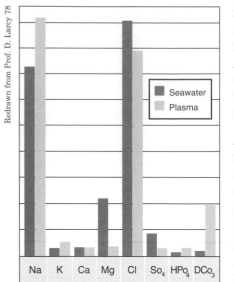

Redrawn from Prof. D. Larcy 78

Seawater
Plasma

Na K Ca Mg Cl So₄ HPo₄ DCo₃

**Chart showing chemical
similarities between plasma
and seawater**

for rheumatism in warm seawater combined with
movement – kinébalneotherapy was born. Bagot also
founded L'Institut Marin de Rockroum in Roscoff on the
Atlantic coast of Brittany, to inaugurate thalassotherapy;
this was originally opened for re-education and cures.
Today the University of Paris medical school operate a
thalassotherapy research centre at Roscoff.

As early as 1904, the French biologist René Quinton
imagined that life began in salt water. He carried out
many experiments to investigate the close chemical
similarities between seawater and blood plasma. Quinton
continued these studies for many years and succeeded in
proving that the chemical pattern of seawater and the
internal human environment are very similar.

In France it is believed that unpolluted seawater also
has a unique anti-bacterial effect due to the presence of
minute plant life (plankton) that keep the sea pure, and
that sea salts contain minute quantities of radioactive
elements that are able to neutralise and balance
radiation.

Although the main component of seawater is sodium
chloride, it is also rich in other minerals and trace
elements such as the chlorides of potassium, magnesium
and calcium, and the sulphates and carbonates of
magnesium and calcium. Near to the coast, it may
contain small quantities of bromine, iodine, boron and
free sulphuric acid. Traces of gold, arsenic, lead, zinc,
copper, silver, strontium, cæsium and rubidium can also
be found.

Seawater cures became very fashionable in Roscoff in
France and Varberg in Sweden during the mid to late
nineteenth century. Thalassotherapy in France, as we
know it today, took off in earnest in 1964 when the
three-times champion cyclist Louison Bobet, and his
brother Jean, opened a huge marine spa at Quiberon

HCB Associates

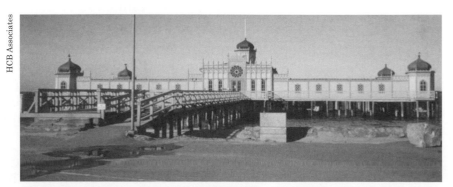

The Bathing House, Varberg, Sweden

The impact of science 13

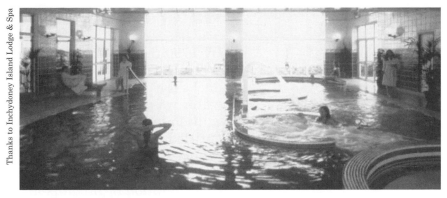

The Thalassotherapy pool, Inchydoney Island Spa, Co. Cork, Republic of Ireland

in Brittany. Bobet had himself benefited from thalassotherapy cures following a severe car accident. After nearly losing both legs, he recovered complete mobility with a regime of physiotherapy in a marine environment (thalassotherapy). Bobet devoted the rest of his life to promoting thalassotherapy.

Recent studies indicate that the salt concentration of the Dead Sea is about 33 per cent – compared to 3 per cent in the Mediterranean. This quality and unique photo (light) biological characteristics are present only in the Dead Sea area. Aristotle (304–322 BC) was the first to tell the world about the wonderful qualities of the Dead Sea: 'very bitter and salty water in which no fish can live and where neither man nor animal can sink'.

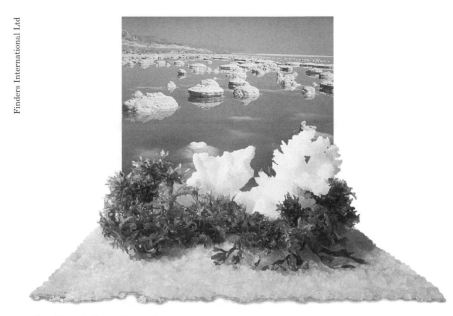

The Dead Sea, Israel

Water and fashion

By 1790 the popularity of water was such that Horace Walpole observed: 'One would think that the English are ducks for they are forever waddling to the waters'. Cold water was so fashionable that doctors began to advise caution in its use. Dr William Buchan compiled a tract entitled, *Cautions Concerning Cold Bathing and Drinking Mineral Waters* in 1786. This was published at the same time as James Makittrick Adair's *Medical Cautions for the Consideration of Invalids* and his *Essays on Fashionable Diseases*, published for the General Hospital in Bath.

Water and fevers

However, the effects of cold water on fevers were being noticed and published, most notably by James Currie, the man who received the publicity and is best remembered for his work. In fact, three men made this important observation – all at about the same time. The first was Dr Wright, later President of the Royal College of Physicians of Edinburgh, who had buckets of cold water thrown over him when he was *en route* from Jamaica in 1777. The treatment was called bucketing and was also used in the spa at Bath. (In England bucketing sometimes meant pouring water through a sponge.) He published his findings nine years later. The second man was Robert Jackson, who noted the effects in 1791, but did not go into print until 1808. He also claimed to have introduced cold bathing to the British army. Dr James Currie, who treated 153 feverish patients over a four-year period in Liverpool, was the third man to commit the cases to print in 1797.

The cold water cure in Europe

The founder of what is now called **hydrotherapy** – the external and internal use of water – was Vincent Priessnitz (1799–1851) the 19-year-old uneducated son of a Silesian farmer in Graefenberg in the Jesenik mountains, in what is now the Czech Republic.

Priessnitz's name is still remembered in European spas today. Run over by a farm cart, he sustained multiple bruises and three fractured ribs. His doctor thought he would never work again, but the young man was determined to live life to the full. He recalled seeing, as a boy, an old man cure diseases in cattle by the external application of cold water. He had also observed injured animals recover from their injuries by bathing in streams

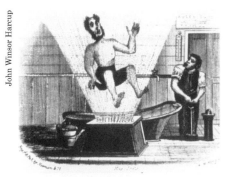

Ascending douche

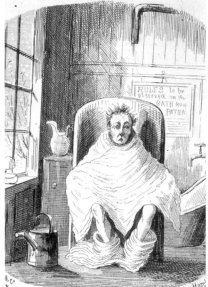

Cartoon of a sitz bath with limb wrapping. Note the 'douche' pipe above the patient which delivered more than 450 litres of cold water onto the naked patient in a matter of seconds.

and pools. It is recorded that, on returning home he persuaded his friends to wet the sheets from his bed and wrap them round his chest, after he had leant against a chair and taken a deep breath to re-align his ribs.

The sheets were soaked again and again with cold water as they dried out. Within ten days he was able to go out and after a year he was back at work and had formulated his regime of the cold water cure, involving wrapping with wet sheets, various cold baths, combined with fresh air, diet and exercise – very similar to some spa treatments and regimes today. This health package was called the Priessnitz cure and the sanatorium in Graefenberg, which he set up in 1829 and where he treated 49 patients, is still in existence today.

By 1842, there were between 40 and 50 hydropathic establishments – the name coined to describe them – in Germany, Hungary, Poland and Russia. Over the first 12 years, 7000 patients, including the crowned heads of Europe, tried the cure.

At Graefenberg, the first bath of the day lasted three minutes, followed by a walk until breakfast. Douches, full and half (or **sitz**) baths, cold wet sheets and rubbings with towels completed the regime. All drugs and alcohol were banned. The bath water was at a temperature of 43–50°F (6–10°C). Priessnitz personally supervised all the treatments, feeling the pulse of his patients and assessing the state of their skin before advising the length of time they were to be immersed in the bath – usually up to eight minutes or 'before the second sensation of cold'.

It did not matter that Priessnitz wrote no books and left no notes for amongst many others who visited Priessnitz were Sir Charles Scudamore, Captain R. T. Claridge and Dr James Wilson who all described the treatments in detail. Sir Charles wrote *A Medical Visit to Graefenberg for the purpose of investigating the water cure treatment in 1843* and realised that Priessnitz inspired in his patients 'the most entire confidence and he extracts implicit obedience', concluding that 'P has no principles of medical knowledge to reason from, beyond those which he has learnt from a long study of nature'.

Sir Charles also noted the temperatures for wet sheet wrapping – 64°F (18°C) for 'very delicate patients', whilst the more robust tolerated 50°F (10°C). Full or plunge baths were as low as 44°F (6.6°C) in the early morning or after dinner. He wrote of the sitz bath or hipbath for 'many types of disorders affecting the parts situated within the male and female pelvis'.

The cold water cure in England

The pioneers of hydrotherapy in England are often cited as Dr James Wilson and Captain Claridge, but the honours should be shared with Dr Weiss, who practised with Priessnitz for 12 years, once treating the future Napoleon III.

Mr C. Von Schlemmer, a pupil of Professor Dr Oertel of Bavaria, claimed to have practised at 'the first hydropathic establishment in England at Ham Common in Surrey'. This was Mr Henry Wright's Allcott House School, where Von Schlemmer had come with his son to learn English. From 1 December 1841 he 'encouraged 40 or 50 persons to take daily cold baths and treated hydropathically, illnesses ranging from measles to croup and other conditions', occurring in the school at that time. He claimed that cold bathing – 'revives and strengthens the nerves and muscles . . . accelerates the circulation of the blood, promotes digestion' and, like so many others, he stressed the need for acclimatisation, declaring that 'delicate patients are prepared for the full bath by tepid baths during the first week or two'.

The following year found Von Schlemmer working as 'sub-director of Gaefenberg House, Stanstead Bury, near Hertford' under Dr Weiss. Gaefenberg House, Stanstead Bury was modelled on the Silesian spa.

It was Dr Thomas Graham of Epsom and Sackville Street, London, who had persuaded Dr Weiss to come to England. Graham appeared to be an expert in treating debility, which he defined as 'want of tone and energy in the nervous system, where patients cannot bear the lightest smell or slightest sound without excessive suffering'. This sounds something like the Chronic Fatigue Syndrome of today. Graham pronounced that the cold water system, 'cautiously employed, will tone the nerves, enable the patient to get out of bed and by degrees be cured'.

Dr James Wilson and Malvern

The story of how Dr James Wilson firmly established the Priessnitz cure in England starts with the doctor's disillusionment with Victorian medicine, where heavy metal poisons and alkaloids, such as opium, were used indiscriminately to the detriment of the patient.

In the 1840s Wilson gave up his practice to work as travelling physician to Lord Farnham, whose fussiness was soon too much for him. He found himself out of work and wandering around Europe. His own health problems eventually led him to the Silesian spa in the Jesenik Mountains, where he stayed for eight months observing Priessnitz at work.

During that time it is recorded that Wilson sat in 500 cold baths, 240 sitz baths, spent 480 hours wrapped in wet sheets and drank 3500 glasses of cold water. One morning he is said to have overdone water ingestion when he consumed 30 glasses before breakfast – 20 was the maximum – thus setting a dubious record. Although Priessnitz never discussed the cure with him – language must have been a significant barrier – Wilson was allowed full access as an observer, an indication of the trust between the two men.

Wilson returned to England, 'filled to the brim with hydropathy' as his friend from student days, Dr James Gully, described him years later. Such was the scepticism of the medical profession in England at that time and subsequently, that Gully was the only colleague who would listen to him.

Fired by Wilson's enthusiasm, the two set out to find 'Graefenberg in England.' Malvern, on the Hereford–Worcester border in the West Midlands, had been a village spa for over a century. The Malvern water, bottled since 1622, was made famous by the analysis in 1757 of Dr John Wall, co-founder of the Worcester Infirmary and the Worcester Porcelain Company. In his experiments and observations of the Malvern Waters, Wall found virtually no dissolved matter present, prompting the wits of the eighteenth century to coin a couplet repeated to this day:

> The Malvern Water says Dr John Wall
> Is famous for containing just nothing at all

This lack of minerals is due to the fact that the core of the Malvern Hills is composed of pre-Cambrian granite, the hardest rock in the world. It is from the deepest part of the earth's crust and water does not dissolve it. Therefore, the water percolating through its billions of tiny fissures does not pick up any minerals.

This village spa on the slopes of the Malvern Hills was ready made for hydropathy when Drs Wilson and Gully arrived by coach from London in the summer of 1842. They soon realised that they had found what they were looking for and leased The Crown Hotel in the centre of Great Malvern and founded Graefenberg House in England. Wilson set about curing a gout-ridden local carrier who made a miraculous recovery, thus ensuring the popularity of the new treatment. Before very long, Malvern was the foremost centre in England for hydropathy for the sick and ailing.

Not all the visitors who came were seriously ill, as Florence Nightingale observed during a visit with her mother in 1848 – 'Malvern has become a highly popular amusement amongst athletic invalids, who have felt the tedium vitae and have those indefinite diseases which a large income and unbounded leisure are so well calculated to produce.' However, in 1857, exhausted by her efforts in the Crimean War and the struggle to complete an important report, she collapsed and fled to Malvern, later confessing 'after my work at the Royal Sanitary Commission . . . I was told that my life was not worth 24 hour's purchase and I knew it too. I owe three years of (not useless) life to the water cure at Malvern'. She went on to live to a ripe old age.

Who was cured

Other famous visitors included an extremely depressed Charles Darwin who, after 16 weeks, felt 'certain that the Water Cure is no quackery' and went back to his home at Down House to write a book about barnacles.

Alfred, Lord Tennyson was, as he put it, 'half cured, half destroyed' by the therapy. However, Mrs Jane Carlyle, who was obviously addicted to drugs, wrote, after a visit with her famous husband Thomas, 'I have not swallowed a pill since I left Malvern!!! I am alive and rather well'.

Author Edward Bulwer Lytton 'threw physic [drugs] to the dogs and went to Malvern'. Here he found 'patients accustomed for half a century to live hard and high, wine-drinkers and spirit-bibbers whom their regular physician has sought in vain to reduce to a daily pint of sherry, here voluntarily resign all potations [sic], after a day or two cease to feel the want of them and reconcile themselves to water as if they had drunk nothing else all their lives'. He also saw 'those who had recourse for years and years to medicine – their potion in the morning, their cordial at noon, their pill before dinner and their narcotic at bedtime – cease to require these aids to life as if by charm'.

Other spectacular cures were claimed by tired and stressed wealthy Victorians who overate and over-drank.

The lifestyle at Malvern was so important that Lytton encapsulated the regime in the words: 'At the Water Cure the whole life is one remedy'. The holistic approach, on which the modern international spa ethos is based, was being used in Malvern more than 150 years ago.

A day in the life of a water cure patient

The day started for the patient with a wake-up call at 5 or 6 a.m. from the bath attendant who wrapped the naked client in cold wet sheets for an hour. A blanket and counterpane placed on top made them resemble an Egyptian mummy.

As the warmth of the body dried out the sheets, a delicious sense of sleep and relaxation crept over the immobile patient. This was followed by a shallow bath, then more water poured over the head and shoulders before the whole body was rubbed down with a coarse towel. This was called a friction rub.

Then, before breakfast, visitors were sent up the hills to drink at every spring using flattened flasks, called Graefenberg flasks. Breakfast was a healthy affair with milk, porridge, cold meat and water, bread, boiled rice and treacle. Later in the morning there were baths in between leisure activities, such as billiards or reading the London papers.

At midday, for those who were fit enough, the ordeal of the douche took place, when cold water from the springs on the hills cascaded 20 feet (6.5 metres) from a pipe 2.5 inches

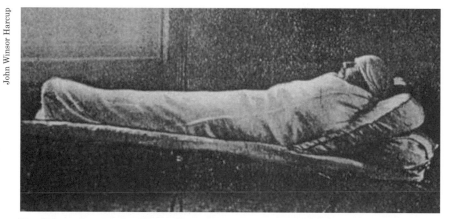

Packing circa 1900 from Metcalf's 'Rise and Fall of Hydrotherapy in England and Scotland'

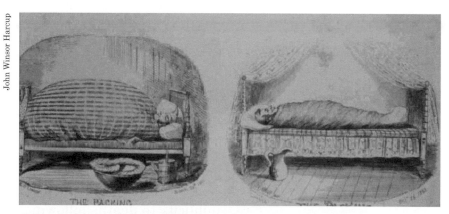

Cartoons of packing with cold wet sheets circa 1850

(6.35 cm) or 3.5 inches (8.9 cm) in diameter onto the patient's naked body at the rate of one hogshead per minute (52.5 imperial gallons or 238 litres). There was a set ritual for receiving the chilled column of water falling 20 feet – first on one side of the shoulder, then on the other, followed by a part of the spine then the whole spine, but never on the head unless the fingers were interlaced over the neck and crown to break the waterfall into a 'delicious shower of foam'. The douche lasted for a minimum of three minutes to a maximum of eight. In three minutes the hapless patient would receive 150 gallons or 682 litres of water.

Other treatments included spinal washing, abdominal compresses, foot and hand baths, the lamp bath (actually a mini Turkish bath where the client sat on a stool swathed in a blanket with a lamp burning underneath him) and a sweating process where the patient was covered by many blankets.

Clever publicity

At the end of their first year in Malvern, Wilson and Gully, who by this time had established separate facilities, leaving Wilson with Graefenberg House, embarked on a clever piece of publicity in the form of a book entitled *The Dangers of the Water Cure*. This stated that it was unwise to take the cure supervised by doctors who were inexperienced in the techniques.

Other risks were 'inadequate investigations and slovenly treatment administered by inexperienced practitioners' and the fact that recovery could be hampered by the ingestion 'of spiced and otherwise stimulating food, alcoholic liquors of any kind and drugs of any sort'.

It was also deemed dangerous to allow 'mental distractions and irritations of business or the passions' to interfere with the healing process. Gully took this to extremes and segregated the sexes in his establishment into two houses – Tudor House for men and Holyrood House for women, linked by what the humorous periodical, *Punch*, dubbed 'The Bridge of Sighs'.

The Dangers of the Water Cure was printed together with a prospectus of their respective establishments that proudly proclaimed that nearly 600 cases had been treated with 'not a single disagreeable result that could be, in any way, attributed to the system of treatment by water'.

There were several attempts over the years to discredit the Water Cure by jealous orthodox practitioners giving adverse publicity to deaths following water treatment, but none was ever proved to have been due to the direct action of cold water. The most vociferous verbal battle on this subject was between Wilson and the Worcester-based Dr Charles Hastings, later Sir Charles, the founder of what became the British Medical Association.

The Dangers of the Water Cure included a prospectus containing a set of propositions to explain the new regime and clothe it in a cloak of scientific respectability, designed to appeal to the middle and upper classes, their market at this time. Proposition number 24 summarised the core of the cure: 'Pure water, pure air, proper diet and regulated exercise, are the great agents in effecting the cure of disease by aiding the natural efforts of the body, through the instrumentality of the nervous system'.

Even surgeons took up the Water Cure. Mr R. J. Culverwell, in his *Hydropathy or the Cold Water Cure as adopted by Vincent Priessnitz*, made a very practical suggestion concerning the best way to brave the low temperature which put so many off the regime – 'it is better to effect the general immersion at once than creep in feet first by degrees'. He also recommended acclimatisation, daily bathing and the use of a 'douche bidet' for home use, which was a sort of ascending douche – what we call a bidet today. This apparatus was said to be beneficial for piles, 'inflammatory and painful attacks of the perineum, loins and affections of the bladder, uterine relaxation and all attendant disappointments'!

The cure spreads throughout Great Britain

By the mid 1800s, Water Cure establishments had sprang up all around Great Britain; there were a number near London at Epsom, Farnham, Harrow, Kingston, Streatham and Tunbridge Wells. Further afield, doctors dispensed their water treatments during the mid-nineteenth century at Cheltenham, Dunstable, Grasmere in the Lake District, Manchester, Umberslade Hall, Ramsgate, Ryde on the Isle of Wight, Cork in Ireland and Aberdeen, Forres, Kirn, and Rothsay in Scotland. The most famous satellite spa of Malvern was Ben Rhydding, near Ilkley in Yorkshire, known as 'The Aesculapian of the North'.

Some spa entrepreneurs

Some spa owners were not doctors, but interested entrepreneurs. The most famous was mill-owner John

Smedley (1803–74), who set-up his well-known Hydro at Matlock Bath and treated 5000 patients in five years. His huge building still commands a lofty site in the town.

Another spa entrepreneur of the time was Richard Beamish, who tried the cure in 1842 and as a result opened an establishment at Prestbury near Cheltenham, with Albert Priessnitz, brother of Vincent, as his 'most able manipulator'. He was enthusiastic about the 'triumphs of hydropathy in the cure of asthma' and believed that 'water relieves weakness' in cases of debility.

The American connection

Gully's book *The Water Cure in Chronic Disease*, published in 1846, appeared in the USA nine months later. The concept of cold water treatment had crept across the Atlantic when the American edition of John Smith's *Curiousities of Common Water* was published in 1723.

Smith wrote for all those who could not afford medical bills. His frontispiece explained: 'That's the best physick [drug] which doth cure our ills without the charge of 'Pothecarie's [apothecarie's or chemist's] Bills'. He extolled the virtues of cold water in 'want of sleep, swoonings and over-active children'. Smith later wrote about some success in treating cholera. American physician Dr Benjamin Rush also found cold water 'a most agreeable and powerful remedy in bilious yellow fever'.

American pioneers

By 1843–44, a Water Cure establishment based on the principles laid down by Priessnitz had been opened in New York City by two of the four founders of the American movement, Drs Joel Shew and R. T. Trall.

By 1848, there were 30 such institutions in nine states. Trall developed hydropathy into a healing philosophy called 'The Philosophy of Medical Science and a system of Hygienic Medication'. This was based on 'the art of healing with the laws of nature'. Water was the central element and could be of 'universal application'. Trall believed that disease was due to impure blood, unhealthy secretions, obstructions to blood flow in capillaries and the excessive or deficient function of various organs. It was this loss of balance in the body which water corrected, with help from the natural forces of air, light, food (diet) and temperature.

Spas in America spread and developed differently from the Water Cure establishments in Europe; they were water playgrounds, demanding little from patients and omitting the key factors of air, exercise and diet. As one observer noted, 'spas had become more a social than a therapeutic episode'. And the hydropathic periodical *Herald of Health* classified the minerals in spa water as drugs and condemned the practice of 'running after sulphur, iodine, iron and other drugged water for health purposes'.

Hydropathic medical schools

The two other prominent figures on the American hydropathic scene were Dr T. L. Nichols and Mary Grove, a hydropath and a health reformer, who became his wife. Grove was mainly self-taught in medicine and claimed to be one of the first women to qualify in medicine, but she was unable to practise in her own right because of sexual discrimination.

In 1851, the couple opened what was said to be the first medical school in the world called The American Hydropathic Institute, based on water cure principles. It lasted only three terms. Trall was more successful with his New York Hydropathic School, which started with 50 students in 1853 and continued, with a name change, for over nine years.

Dr and Mrs Nichols finally fled the American Civil War and came to England, eventually settling in Great Malvern, where Mary wrote her feminist book *A Woman's Work in Water Cure and Sanitary Education* (1874). In it she argued for more female physicians, the right of a woman to choose a doctor of her own sex and a radical change in attitudes to women's diseases, pointing out that the causes were often due to ignorance and therefore were avoidable.

Grove recommended the ascending douche – the modern bidet – in contrast to the widely used descending one, and syringing for vaginal discharges. She opposed the use of warm baths on the grounds that they were too comforting!

Summing up her time in Malvern, she wrote: 'I think that my greatest success has been in teaching persons to cure themselves, so that they will neither require to come to me nor any other physician'.

Decline and hygiene

The heyday of the American water cure lasted until the late 1850s when establishments appeared in attractive rural areas reached by railroad, stagecoach or steamboat.

Consequent over-expansion, business depression and the Civil War led to a decline in numbers, but at least three dozen survived. However, the end of fighting brought radical changes in America and the establishments became hygienic institutions, with water no longer seen as the principal agent.

American hot springs

The most famous of these hygienic institutions is Sarotoga Springs in New York, but the Hot Springs of Arkansas, Safety Harbour in Florida, Calistoga in the Napa Valley and the White Sulphur Springs of West Virginia have all survived to the present day. Sarotoga, however, is the grandest example of American spa culture. The name is a Mohawk Indian word meaning 'the place of the medicine waters of the great spirit'.

Its main hot water source is the High Dome Spring, so-called because of its domed structure, constructed of mineral deposits, which was discovered in 1767. Six years later, Dick Schouten constructed a log cabin next to the spring. In the following year, John Arnold turned it into the first US pleasure resort. It was rebuilt in 1826 as a village, in an architectural style reminiscent of a European spa.

The Boyes Hot Springs near Calistoga dates from 1895 and was redeveloped and renamed in 1928 as the Sonoma Mission Inn and Spa. Towards the end of the twentieth century, it was re-equipped to give body treatments such as massage, beauty treatments and fitness features.

Science, cornflakes and biscuits

Dr William Winternitz, a lecturer in hydropathy at Vienna Medical School, is known for his research into the physiology of water immersion and the scientific aspects of the cold water cure. He became known as 'The Father of Scientific Hydrotherapy'. He opened a clinic and an Institute of Hydrotherapy near Vienna in 1861 and attracted students from all over the world, including the United States.

One American student was Dr John Harvey Keith Kellogg (1852–1943), who practised at Battle Creek Sanatorium for 46 years from 1876. Kellogg, the hydropathist is now forgotten, but the family name is still world famous through his brother, W(illie) K(eith) Kellogg, who invented a process of rolling and baking corn to make a nourishing breakfast cereal for the patients at Battle Creek during the

1890s. In a similar vein, Dr William Oliver, in the early 1700s, invented the Bath Oliver biscuit to help visitors digest the waters of Bath. Both these foodstuffs are still available today.

A famous Bavarian priest

Following in the footsteps of Priessnitz was a very popular therapist, Father Sebastian Kneipp, a German priest from Bavaria. Said to be a 'simple man of the people', he studied medicine and accidentally found himself involved in hydropathy by curing a village of cholera in 1854.

His establishment in Bad Worishofen, opened in 1889, relied on wet sheets and cold baths where the whole body was immersed for a minimum of 30 seconds and a maximum of three minutes. There were also limb baths, vapour and shower baths.

Fr Kneipp preached that cold baths 'refresh, vivify the whole organism' and ' the shorter the bath, the better the effect'. His book, *My Water Cure* (published in 1886), describes how he 'hardened' his patients by making them 'walk barefoot on wet grass, snow, stones or in cold water'. The Kneipp cure – the **Kniepp Kur System** – was also a package of health measures, like that of Priessnitz, but in addition, included lifestyle change and plant therapy.

Kneipp attracted a large following in Europe and influenced the development of the Nature Cure movement of the early twentieth century. The Kneipp cure is still widely practised in spas today, especially treading in cold water and the utilisation of plant therapy. **Kniepp baths** are herbal or mineral baths of varying temperatures used in combination with diet and exercise.

The rise of natural methods

The Nature Cure movement gained momentum following the popularity of the health packages of Priessnitz and Kneipp and gave rise to a complementary medical system still practised today. Dr John Scheel of New York first used the name, **naturopathy**, in 1895. The following year Benedict Lust, a follower of Kneipp, founded The American School of Naturopathy in New York.

The natural remedies used in the treatment were wholesome foods, herbs, air and water, assisted by physical procedures such as massage and manipulation. Surgery and drugs were avoided. The aim of this regime was to assist the body to overcome disease. Dr John Kellogg (see page 24) was a convert, as were many others.

Henry Lindlahr, in his *Philosophy of Natural Therapeutics* (1918), set out the argument that, as the body has the ability to heal itself by mending broken bones and filling wounds, it is capable of curing other conditions.

Massage, physiotherapy and water

The Greeks practised massage, or rubbing as it was called, to tone the body. Hippocrates was said to be an expert on this subject and to have advised a daily scented bath and massage in order to keep healthy. The Romans were massaged in their homes or at the public baths by doctors, their assistants or trainers.

However, it was not until 1500 years later that massage became fully accepted by the medical profession when the French Surgeon Ambroise Pare (1517–91) graded rubbing into strengths – gentle, medium or vigorous. In England, a surgeon named John Grosvenor (1742–1823) used massage to treat diseased joints. Subsequently, modern massage techniques (also known as **Swedish massage**) were developed by a Swedish physiologist, Per Henrick Ling (1776–1839), who also devised a system of exercises known as Swedish Remedial Gymnastics. Massage for rehabilitation was devised by a Dutch physician, Johan Mezgner (1839–1909), and gained worldwide acceptance.

By the end of the nineteenth century, nurses were being encouraged to train and use massage under the supervision of a doctor. A group formed themselves into the Society of Trained Masseuses, which in 1920 joined the Institute of Massage and Remedial Exercise. Given a Royal Charter in recognition of their valuable work done during the First World War, this became the Chartered Society of Massage and Medical Gymnastics. Exercises in water became part of rehabilitation programmes used by the trained masseuses, whose organisation went on to become the Chartered Society of Physiotherapy in 1943.

In the USA, the 1920s saw the development of the Hubbard tank, in which patients could perform remedial exercises in water. L. W. Hubbard (1857–1938) was an American orthopaedic surgeon who specialised in treating cases of polio.

In the twenty-first century, hydrotherapy is used in hospitals worldwide by physiotherapists specially trained in the treatment of injuries, to help brain-damaged children and to aid recovery from post-operative conditions and strokes.

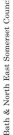

Bath & North East Somerset Council

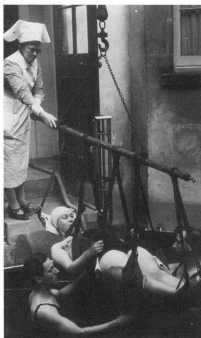

Patient lowered into exercise pool, hot baths, Bath, UK

Water and World Wars

During both World Wars, spas were actively involved in the treatment of the wounded and those invalided out of the services. The conditions treated included rheumatism, joint and muscle injuries, war wounds, neuroses and shell shock, as well as neurasthenia (a psychological disorder, characterised by fatigue, feelings of inadequacy and psycho-somatic symptoms). This created a massive workload and the main spas involved were Bath, Buxton, Cheltenham, Droitwich and Harrogate in England, Llandrindod in Wales and Stathpeffer in Scotland. Red Cross treatment centres were set up in Brighton and London, using sites at Holland Park, Great Portland Street and Shepherds Bush, where there was a special hydrological unit.

There was a lack of interest amongst the medical profession in rheumatic diseases at this time and it fell to those in spas to stimulate research and debate in the subject, through organisations such as the British Spa Federation (formed in 1917) and the Section of Balneology and Climatology of the Royal Society of Medicine, which took over the British Balneology and Climatology Society of 1896 in 1909.

In 1950, L'Academie de Médecine in France set out the principles for controlling the use of sea and spring water in the treatment of an illness. Adrien Barthelemy of Toulouse in France bought up a forgotten spa, Molitg-les-Bains, a hot, sulphurous spring where algae flourish. Barthelemy established the 'Chaine Thermale de Soleil' at the Maison du Thermalisme in Paris.

In Britain, the financial constraints of both wars meant that little or no money was invested in spas during or after the hostilities. They consequently became run-down and were unable to meet the challenges of the twentieth century, which saw the advent of the National Health Service, and the technological revolution in medicine with the switch to powerful drug treatments and amazing advances in surgical and diagnostic techniques. Both doctors and politicians argued for evidence-based medicine, where proof of efficacy was needed in order for a treatment to be accepted. The holistic approach, with its reliance on natural healing and the avoidance of many drugs, condemned spas to the sidelines.

In the UK, the traditional healing spas were regarded as relics of the past by this new breed of doctor, while in Europe their cultural worth and popularity were maintained.

Water in the space age

After the Second World War, the importance of water immersion received a boost in the USA when NASA scientists were looking for a way to simulate weightlessness in space. They found that the nearest situation on Earth to being in space was immersion up to the neck in water at body temperature.

Over several decades, Murray Epstein researched HOWI (Head Out of Water Immersion) in the United States, noting the effects, especially on the kidneys, and working out the chemical changes which occurred as a result.

Cold water research

In the 1990s, Professor Vijay Kakkar, director of the London Thrombosis Research Institute, worked out a regime of TRHT (Thermo-Regulatory Hydrotherapy), where volunteers were acclimatised to cold water, by reducing the temperature and increasing the time of HOWI over a period of 80 days.

Kakkar found that a number of physiological changes resulted in the immune, cardiovascular, hormonal and renal systems of the body. The body's immune response was activated as if challenged by an infective agent, such as a virus or bacterium, and that thyroid, heart function and renal output were stimulated. These were all beneficial effects. One unexpected finding was that cold water causes the release of a number of proteins, which block the clotting mechanism and thin the blood. It had previously been thought that cold caused blood clotting. However, it seems that nature has a protective mechanism ready for when we are chilled.

This research has vindicated the cold water regimes advocated down the centuries and shown that Charles Darwin was right in his assessment that 'The Water Cure is no quackery', despite the bizarre nature of some of the treatments, when put into the context of the treatments available at the time.

Promoting spas today

Steps to promote spas began in earnest with the formation of the European Spa Association (ESPA) in 1995. This sprang from earlier attempts by the British Spas Federation (BSF) and the German Spa Association (DBV) in response to an initiative by the Federation

Internationale du Thermalisme et du Climatisme (FITEC) to form a European association, which would influence the EU in Brussels. Membership was initially confined to EU member states.

The aims were to promote spas by exchange of ideas, publishing a map of spas, educating doctors in spa medicine, harmonising training, identifying standards and intensifying spa research. At the time of writing, FITEC and the French, Italian and Russian spa associations are not in ESPA.

The International Spa Association (ISPA) was formed in the USA in 1991 and is composed largely of those involved in the spa industry – owners, operators, managers, equipment manufacturers and product houses rather than doctors and scientists. It has since spread worldwide, although it is still US driven. A European chapter was started in 1996 and an Asia-Pacific chapter in 1998; both were dissolved in September 2002. ISPA continues to seek to further the interests of the spa industry throughout the world, where spas are meeting the challenges of the twenty-first century in the quest for fitness, well-being and by providing facilities for health tourism.

In 2004, the British Spas Federation, formed in 1917 to promote the interests of the spa towns of the UK, changed its name to The Spa Business Association to become an inclusive organisation for all those employed in, investing in, or supplying the spa industry in the UK and Ireland. The stated mission of the SpaBA is to provide 'one voice' for the spa industry, its collective interests in government, in the media, and to all the customers. Anyone working in the spa business can apply for membership, whether as a spa operator, a supplier of equipment or services, or as an individual working in the industry or as a student member.

In 2002, Rostock, on the Baltic coast, saw the first European Congress for Thalassotherapy, which sought to define and promote seaside spas.

A unique spa country

Iceland, with huge amounts of geothermal water freely available, appeared on the spa scene in 1955 when Dr Jònas Krisjànsson founded the Health and Rehabilitation Clinic of the Nature Heath Association of Iceland (HNLFI), which treats a wide range of illnesses from arthritis to breast cancer, obesity and stress. Patients are residential for up to four weeks and have a variety of treatments, including water and volcanic mud baths, an organic diet and exercise.

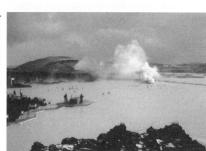

John Winsor Harcup

The blue lagoon, Grindawik, Iceland on the outskirts of Reykjavik

A byproduct of the geothermal water is the famous Blue Lagoon, so called because of the blue green algae which live in the silica-laden water. The condition of patients with psoriasis is vastly improved by immersion in the milky blue water.

With low pollution levels, few trees in the volcanic and glacial landscape, and a different pollen season from Western Europe, Iceland is becoming a haven for asthma and hay fever sufferers. In the capital Reykjavik, there are more spas per capita than anywhere else in the world. Since the year 2000, it has been called Reykjavik Spa City. Most of Reykjavik's thermal pools are outdoors and used all the year round. Each features 'hot pots' which are tubs, unique to Iceland, some three metres in diameter with temperatures ranging from 37–42°C (98–111°F) and used in ascending temperatures. Enjoyed in conjunction with saturated steam baths, hot pots effectively revitalise and relax the body.

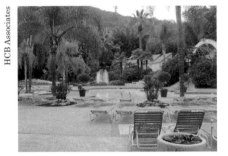

HCB Associates

Glen Ivy Hot Springs Spa, California, USA

American 'super spas'

The past 40 years have witnessed the rise of American 'super spas' which preserve the privacy of the individual and effectively cocoon clients from the outside world. They serve a variety of needs from weight-reduction to pampering and 'stress-busting'. Vastly different from the 'Old World' spas, they are extremely popular and there are now over 200 of them.

Spas in Asia

Bathing in mineral springs is an ancient tradition in Japan. There are over 2000 hot, cold and warm springs and, like the Roman soldiers, the Samurai and military noblemen frequented them. Atami, Shuzenji, Suwa and Dogo are some of the oldest. Spiritual beings, known as *kami*, were thought to live in the medicinal waters, giving spiritual vision and guidance.

Kyushu University in Beppu founded the Balneotherapy Institute in 1931 and began a scientific research programme on the springs. By 1955, there were over 90 medical facilities in the mineral springs locations, using water to treat rheumatism, diseases of the stomach, intestines, liver, skin disease and gout, as well as offering rehabilitation.

The development of the modern Asian spa market as a tourism phenomenon is relatively young, with the opening of three major spas in Thailand in 1993.

The healing philosophies of traditional Chinese medicine

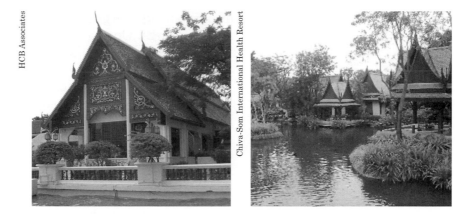

HCB Associates

Chiva-Som International Health Resort

**The Oriental Hotel and Spa,
Bangkok, Thailand**

**Chiva-Som International Health
Resort, Hua Hin, Thailand**

(TCM) have been adopted by many Asian spas and,
although the therapies may vary from country to country
due to the availability of ingredients used in the
treatments, the concepts are the same. The focus of Chinese
practice is individuality, where the client/guest will receive
a unique combination of therapies, working with the body's
energy system to drive the entire physical organism. The
treatment programme is based upon what are known as the
'Three Treasures', which are the various elements that
interact within the body.

1. *energy* – or life force, called **Qi** or **Chi**

2. *jing* – the essence which governs vitality and longevity

3. *shen* – the mind or spirit, responsible for consciousness
    and mental ability.

TCM (traditional Chinese medecine) utilises a number of
therapies:

- herbal medicine
- tui na
- qi gong and tai ji
- acupuncture (zhen fa)
- moxibustion (jiu fa)
- **acupressure**
- **reflexology**.

Asian physicians developed the sophisticated diagnostic
skill of taking the pulse to determine the patient's physical
state whilst they were fully clothed, as it was considered
indecent to touch the body of a person of the opposite sex
(the Wellness Library, London).

The Oriental in Bangkok and the Banyan Tree in Phuket
were the first examples of spa resorts specialising in the art

of pampering the guest in luxurious and exotic surroundings. Chang Mai, Phuket, Pattaya and Samui in Thailand developed similar resort/hotel spas (see Chapter 7, page 198 for definitions) soon after. Chiva-Som at Hua Hin is Thailand's only destination spa – *Condé Nast Traveller* rated it 'best in category' for 2002. The St Carlos in Bangkok is Thailand's only true medical spa. Chiva-Som does offer some medical treatments, such as echocardiography (diagnosing cardiovascular disease), physiotherapy, cleansing diet, blood testing and nutritional analysis.

Spas, in combination with MICE (meetings, incentives, conferences and exhibitions), are the fastest growing trends in Asia's travel industry.

The Thai spa market has overtaken Bali's, with the day spa market for casual visitors rapidly growing and competing with hotels. Thailand has a rich tradition of massage, herbal and steam treatments, using indigenous ingredients to create exotic therapies. Seventy per cent of all treatments in Thai spas are massage-based. Now that an international market has been opened, body wraps, hydrotherapy, floral baths, hair and beauty treatments as well as mind and body therapies such as meditation, **tai chi**, **yoga** and acupuncture are offered, often using locally produced products based upon Thai herbal medicine. Thai spas aim to give their clients a 'feel-good factor', with plenty of 'hands on' treatments and only limited use of mechanical equipment, which is reserved more for the beauty salon.

International spa operators and consultants now own growing numbers of spa centres and bring expertise and experience from a long tradition of spa culture. At the start of the twenty-first century, the main spa operators include:

- Mandara
- Banyan Tree and Angsana
- Six Senses
- Central Hotels and Resorts (Centara)
- Dusit Group (Devarana; *devarana* is an ancient Sanskrit word for 'garden found at the gate of Heaven').

Some groups offer branded spa menus and products, trained managers and therapists, apprenticeship schemes, and uniformed staff; others prefer to create a unique image. Most operators have in-house training programmes ensuring that their brand is understood and carried through at every level to the highest standards.

Asia is known for service. The Banyan Tree, Mandara Spas and Chiva-Som operate their own schools with foreign expertise being brought in for specialist training. Traditional Thai massage is taught at Wat Po, near the Royal Palace in Bangkok. A 20-hour, 10-week, government-approved and supervised course costs $3,800 barts (£63.00) in the year 2000. The Thai labour department is keen to establish formal training in the Thai treatments and is working together with the Thai Spa Association to draft regulations and standards for the Asian spa industry and to offer accreditation to spa members.

The role of water today

In the UK, water is now used in medicine for the treatment of rheumatic diseases and rehabilitation after accidents, sports injuries or surgery as well as for relaxation in spas and in centres of well-being. On the continent, spas are still very much part of the culture of several countries and are used in the treatment of a wide variety of medical conditions. Worldwide, water is used for fitness, well-being and that elusive 'feel-good' factor.

So relaxing are the various types of water treatments that they are widely used in spas. Recent research has shown that improvements in quality of life and increased function after spa and water therapy treatments persists for weeks or sometimes months. This is a major factor in the holistic spa experience and accounts for the seemingly insatiable demand. The continued popularity of water throughout the centuries is evidence of its effectiveness and modern science is now providing proof for this.

References

British Spas Federation, 1930, *The Spas of Great Britain*, official handbook of the British Spas Federation, BSF, Bath.

Coley, Noel, 1979, '"Cures without Care", "Chymical Physicians" and mineral waters in seventeenth century English medicine', *Medical History*, 23, 191–214.

Groutier, Alev. E., 1992, *Taking the Waters*, Abbeville Press, New York.

Harcup, John W., 1992, *The Malvern Water Cure*, Winsor Fox Photos, Malvern.

Hembry, Phyllis, 1990, *The English Spa 1560–1815*, Athlone Press, London.

Kakkar, Professor V., 1994, personal communication and *The European*, 23 and 30 September.

Kellaway, G.A. (ed.), 1991, *Hot Springs of Bath*, Bath City Council, Bath.

Porter, Roy (ed.), 1990, *The Medical History of Waters and Spas*, Medical History Supplement, no. 10 (contains Ralph Jackson's monograph).

Rosser, Mo, 1996, *Body Massage*, Hodder & Stoughton, London.

The Shorter Oxford English Dictionary on Historical Principles, 1977, Oxford University Press, Oxford.

Thomson, W.A.R., 1978, *Spas that Heal*, Adam & Charles Black, London.

Turner, E.S., 1967, *Taking the Cure*, Michael Joseph, London.

Wechsberg, Joseph, 1979, *The Lost World of the Great Spas*, Harper & Row, New York.

Weiss, Harry and Howard Kemble, 1967, *The Great American Water-Cure Craze*, The Past Times Press, New Jersey, Trenton.

The physical properties of water

2

Water and life

All life is dependent on water. The average human body is composed of 60 per cent water by weight, although the range is between 40–70 per cent for an adult. A foetus in the womb, developing in an aquatic environment, contains 95 per cent water. Babies 'dry out' after delivery, when their water content drops to 85 per cent. The adult proportion of 60 per cent is attained around puberty.

It is thought that all life was formed in an aquatic environment, sometimes called the primal sea. Life still exists in a watery environment, the cells of the human body contain intracellular fluid and are surrounded by extracellular fluid. There is a resemblance between seawater and extracellular fluid in that the same chemical constituents, minerals and trace elements, are found in each. However, the concentrations of these constituents in seawater and extracellular fluid are different. For example the concentration of salt (NaCl) in extracellular fluid is 0.9 per cent compared with 3 per cent in seawater.

Water in the 'body compartments'

Extracellular fluid is the watery environment in which cells function and amounts to 20 per cent of body weight or 14 litres in the average human. Its principal chemical is common salt (NaCl). *Interstitial fluid* surrounds each cell in the form of a gel only one or two molecules thick. This accounts for 3.5 litres of the total 14 litres of the extracellular fluid in the average body. The lymphatic circulatory system prevents the accumulation of excess interstitial fluid and is as widespread as the blood circulation. The lymph accounts for another 3.5 litres of fluid. *Intracellular fluid* fills each cell. Potassium (K+), in the form of a proteinate, a form of protein, is the most important constituent within the cells.

About 1 litre of secretions is always present in the gastrointestinal tract where fluid may be secreted or absorbed quickly as necessary. Up to 10 litres are produced as saliva, gastric juices, bile and intestinal juices every day.

Water balance

Correct hydration is important for the function and stability of cells. Dehydration (lack of water) or overhydration (too much water) decrease cell function. To maintain the correct balance, the membrane covering the cell allows water and various salts of sodium and potassium to pass through it. This is controlled by the so-called 'sodium pump' which is, in reality, an enzyme, sodium-potassium ATPase. This enzyme expels sodium ions from the cell, equal to the number that enter the cell, along what is called an 'electrochemical gradient'. This balances the chemical content of the cell.

The sodium pump over-rides the normal function of osmosis, whereby chemical ions diffuse from a more concentrated solution to a less concentrated one through the semi-permeable membrane of the cell wall to equalise the concentrations on both sides of the membrane.

Trauma and water intoxication

Cell damage (or trauma) from whatever cause, decreases the activity of this enzyme, allowing sodium ions to flood in by osmosis. The result is overhydration and cell destruction.

Though essential to life, too much water can, paradoxically, lead to convulsions and death. This phenomenon of water intoxication is unusual as the human brain has a built-in mechanism to stop the voluntary ingestion of too much water. However, drugs such as ecstasy can switch off this protective mechanism.

The properties of water

Molecular weight

A molecule of water is composed of two hydrogen atoms and one oxygen atom, written as H_2O. The atomic weight of hydrogen is 1 and oxygen 16. Therefore the molecular weight of water is 18. This is a comparatively low value. Because of its low weight, water is able to cross every biological membrane. Hence the description of 'the universality of water'.

The properties of mineral water

The minerals in water also alter its properties. Not only is water a solvent but, depending upon its mineral content, it possesses detergent properties, reduces inflammation (anti-inflammatory) and decreases itching (anti-pruitic). Water with a high salt (sodium chloride) and/or high sulphur content has anti-bacterial and anti-fungal properties. Sulphur also affects skin cell metabolism and is useful in certain skin conditions such as psoriasis and acne.

Minerals and trace elements in water

The following minerals and trace elements are essential to the well-being of the human body:

- *Calcium (Ca)*: Essential for growth and the maintenance of healthy bones and teeth. Important in nerve function, muscle contraction and blood clotting.
- *Magnesium (Mg)*: Promotes enzyme activity, healthy bones and teeth and the correct functioning of muscles, nerves, the metabolic system and the body's use of vitamins B1 and B12.
- *Potassium (K+)*: Essential, with sodium, to maintain the fluid balance of the body. It is also vital for nerve and muscle function.
- *Sodium (Na)*: Works in the same way as potassium, but an excess can cause swelling of the tissues and high blood pressure.
- *Sodium chloride (NaCl)*: A 5 per cent solution relaxes muscles, stimulates the micro-circulation of skin and deeper tissues, benefits the skin metabolism and sensitises the skin to the benefits of UV light (e.g. in the treatment of psoriasis).

A chart of thermal water displayed in the Thermal Spa at the Hotel Habakuk, Maribor, Slovenia

- *Iron (Fe)*: Essential for the production of haemoglobin, the oxygen carrier of the blood; a deficiency causes anaemia and depression of the immune system.
- *Manganese (Mn)*: Required in the control of growth and the functioning of enzymes, nerves and muscles.
- *Sulphur (S)*: Required in the manufacture of protein, healthy hair, nails and skin.
- *Iodine (I)*: Essential for the production of metabolic hormones by the thyroid gland.
- *Bromine (Br)*: Necessary for cell metabolism and natural repair processes.
- *Chlorine (Cl)*: Important in cell metabolism, and the regulation of the acid and alkaline balance of the cells and the blood.

The physical states of water

Water as a biological fluid (this excludes ice, which is incompatible with life), is present in the body either in a solid state, or *gel*, or in a liquid state, or *sol*. The gel exists as extracellular fluid, which surrounds individual cells and forms a gelatinous lattice framework, giving stability and shape to body tissue. The sol or liquid is present in humans as blood, saliva, sweat and tears. In whichever state the water exists in the body, its molecular mobility and permeability remain the same.

Water as a solvent

Water dissolves virtually everything. It can be described as a universal solvent. Almost all the molecules encountered in life are soluble in water.

Water conserves heat

Water can absorb large amounts of heat (or calories) with little or no temperature change. This enables human beings to maintain a stable internal or core temperature, despite differing external temperatures. This ability has allowed mankind to live in diverse extremes of temperature throughout the world, from hot dry deserts to humid tropical rainforests to the cold Arctic regions.

A stable or steady core temperature state is essential for the body's complicated chemical processes that are taking place continuously.

Mechanical effects of water

The most important effect of immersion in water is the Principle of Relative Density, discovered by a Greek mathematician, Archimedes (*c*.287–212 BC). He famously discovered this in his bath and is said to have been so excited that he ran down the street, naked, shouting 'Eureka', meaning 'I've found it'. He realised that when a body is immersed in water it experiences an upward force equal to the weight of water displaced.

The density of water depends on the amount of minerals dissolved in it. The more chemicals there are in the water, the denser it becomes and the greater is the upward force. The relative density of water is set at a ratio of one. This means that any object with a density of less than one will float, and objects with a density greater than one will sink. The adult human body has a relative density of 0.97. This ratio varies with age and the deposition of fat. A fatter adult has a relative density of about 0.86, which is also the ratio for a young child. This explains why certain age groups and body shapes find it easier to float than others.

Each part of the body has a different relative density; the upper limbs are usually less dense than the lower ones which explains why, in water, legs tend to sink and arms tend to float.

Certain illnesses and disabilities alter the density of parts of the body and this must be taken into account in any water treatment involving immersion, whether partial or HOWI (Head Out of Water Immersion).

The effect of hydrostatic pressure

Hydrostatic pressure is another essential factor in bathing and water treatments. The Law of Pascal (1623–62) states that when a body is immersed in a fluid, the pressure exerted on it is equal at a constant depth and is exerted equally in a horizontal direction at any level. This means that the sideways pressure of the fluid on an immersed body is equal on all surfaces at a certain depth. The pressure increases with depth and with increased density of the fluid.

For example, in order to reduce swelling in the lower limbs, they should be immersed in water as deeply as possible. During immersion fluid from the limbs is transferred to the thorax. This input stimulates the kidneys and in turn increases fluid output (*diuresis*) from the body. It has been shown by researchers that immersion for one hour increases water excretion by 50 per cent.

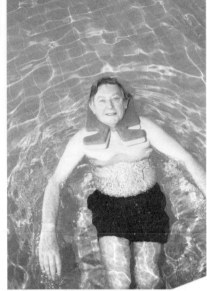

©Phil Pickin

**Droitwich Brine Spa,
Worcestershire, UK**

Body weight in water

A body experiences a sensation of weightlessness in water due to a combination of the upward effects of buoyancy and the sideways effects of hydrostatic pressure. The denser the water, the greater is this feeling of weightlessness. It is therefore easier to float in seawater than tap water.

The Dead Sea in Israel and at Droitwich Spa (Worcestershire, UK) contain so much brine (approximately 10 times the amount of salt than in seawater), that complete weightlessness is possible. Total weightlessness is a unique and unforgettable experience.

Because of the density of the water, performing exercises and walking are easier to do than they are in air, hence the importance of rehabilitation in water after surgery, stroke or sports injury. Immersion also helps to smooth out clumsy, jerky movements at as low a depth as practical.

Balance in water

The Principle of Metacentrics in Hydrostatics was discovered by Bougier (1690–1758) and states that when a body is immersed in water it comes under the influence of two opposing forces: *gravity* and *buoyancy*.

Buoyancy acts in an upward direction, whereas gravity acts downwards. When both these forces are equal and acting in opposite directions, the body is balanced and still. When the forces of buoyancy and gravity are unequal and not strictly in opposing directions, rotational movement occurs. This continues until the forces are equal and acting directly opposite one another.

Water flow

Reynolds (1849–1912) stipulated that there were two types of flow: *laminar* and *turbulent*. Laminar flow produces an even pattern of streamlined molecules, while turbulent flow is uneven, rapid and random, containing eddies and return flows. Working in water can be made more difficult by a transition from laminar to turbulent activity and may affect a disabled person in water.

Other work by Prandtl (1875–1912) described the flow of fluid past a body, where a layer of liquid lies close to the surface of the body. The velocity of this liquid adjacent to the boundary is so slow as to be virtually still and is called the boundary layer. The relevance of this to hydrotherapy is in getting out of the water and it is important for the disabled.

The movement of water is greatest in the centre of a pool and there is little or no movement at the edge, except by the water entry and exit pipes. Clients should be taught and supervised in the technique of getting out of pools, especially if they are disabled. There is a danger of being dragged back into the water, if the exit is clumsy.

Bow wave effect

This is an increase of pressure ahead of the direction of movement due to the column or mass of water in front of the moving body.

Turbulence in water

This is the movement and eddies which occur behind an object moving through water. The amount of turbulence, which occurs with any movement, depends on the speed of movement; eddies only occur at higher speeds. The theorem of Bernoulli (1700–82) concerned the turbulence and the energy of a particle of water at any moment. The total energy of the particle is the sum of its three energies: pressure, potential and kinetic.

The therapist can use this fact to assist or resist movements in water. Therapists should learn how to move safely in water so as not to create turbulence and cause a loss of balance in those being treated. Dealing with the effects of turbulence requires co-ordination and balance, which should be taught as part of a treatment programme.

The drag effect

The energy from the eddies in turbulence spreads out, reducing the pressure; the greater the speed of movement the lower the pressure. The change in pressure creates a drag effect, as an object will always be drawn from an area of high pressure to an area of lower pressure.

The combination of a bow wave in front of a moving body, the turbulence behind it, together with the weight of the water being moved ahead and the tendency for water to adhere or stick to the human body (friction), all contribute to the drag effect.

Physiological changes during immersion in water

The changes that occur in the human body on immersion in water affect the cardiac, circulatory, immune, renal, respiratory systems.

Cardiac effects

During immersion, the hydrostatic pressure exerted on the body causes a shift of blood from the extremities, especially the legs, to the chest where it accumulates in the heart and great blood vessels. This occurs within a matter of minutes.

This effect takes place faster in cold water because the skin circulation shuts down rapidly and approximately 700 ml of blood, or the equivalent of a bottle of wine, is redistributed and returned to the heart. Research has shown that this increases the stroke volume of the heart (the amount of blood ejected by the left ventricle at each contraction) by 35 per cent during thermoneutral (body temperature) immersion.

The heart rate is increased in hot and thermoneutral water and slowed in cold water. In some studies, blood pressure has remained the same, in others the systolic blood pressure shows an increase, more pronounced in cold and hot water than in thermoneutral water. Muscle blood flow increases in hot and neutral temperatures. Hot water induces vasodilatation in the skin's blood vessels.

Soft tissues

Warm water causes muscle relaxation and also has an analgesic effect, though this is not as marked as with cold water. Research has also shown that natural painkillers in the body, such as beta-endorphins, are increased by mineral waters.

Renal system

The hydrostatic pressure exerted on the body's surface increases with every centimetre increment of water depth, resulting in blood being forced from the lower limbs to the heart and chest cavity.

Some researchers have concluded from their work that there is a shift from interstitial fluid to extracellular fluid, with an increase of plasma volume. As a result, the kidneys are stimulated to increase the production of urine and more toxins and waste products are removed. The effect on the kidneys is most noticeable in cold water because of the shut down in the circulation of blood to the skin, as already described.

Respiratory system

Hydrostatic pressure pressing on the chest wall and the influx of blood into the chest cavity as above alters the mechanics of breathing and pulmonary function. There is a decrease in the vital capacity (the volume of air a person can forcibly breathe out after full inhalation) of the lungs, compensated by an increase in capacity during inhalation.

Endocrine system

Immersion in water produces a temporary release and increase of the body's growth hormone. Circulating **cortisol** levels are raised in both hot and cold water and this produces a feeling of euphoria or the 'feel good' factor. The thyroid produces more of the hormone thyroxine, and this increases the metabolic rate of the body.

Immune system

Hot and neutral water immersion stimulate the immune system, but the effect is more marked in cold water with the increased production of CD4 T-cell lymphocytes – the killer white blood cells activated by our immune system.

Other affects include a decrease in the viscosity of the synovial fluid in joints at thermoneutral temperatures which is beneficial for many conditions. Cold water and neutral water have an anti-inflammatory effect on the skin.

Nervous system

Water treatments are beneficial for anxiety and stress conditions because they are extremely relaxing. Temperatures below body temperature, as in a plunge pool, are stimulating, but immersion for longer than 2 minutes surprisingly causes relaxation. The use of a plunge pool for short periods of time can therefore be beneficial in the treatment of depression.

All the physiological phenomena just described are independent of the chemical content and concentration of the water in the spa. In other words, they will apply, whatever type of spa water is being used.

References

Berry, M., R. McMurray and V. Katz, 1989, 'Pulmonary and ventilatory responses to pregnancy, immersion and exercise', *American Physiological Society*, **66**(2), 857–62.

Bonde-Petersen, Flemming, Lone Schultz-Pedersen and Nils Dragsted, 1992, 'Peripheral and central blood flow in man during cold, thermoneutral, and hot water immersion', *Aviation, Space and Environmental Medicine*, May, 346–50.

Campion, Margaret Reid (ed.), 1998, *Hydrotherapy, Principles and Practice*, Butterworth/Heinemann, London.

Epstein, Murray, 1992, 'Renal effects of head-out water immersion in humans: a 15 year update', *American Physiological Society*, 72/3, 563–612.

Franchimont, P. and J. Leconte, 1983, 'Hydrotherapy-mechanisms and indications', *Pharmacology and Therapeutics*, 20, 79–93.

Ghersetich, I. and Lolti, T.M. 1996, 'Immunology of mineral water spas', *Clinics in Dermatology*, 14, 563–6.

Hong, S., P Cerretell, J. Cruz and H. Rahn, 1969, 'Mechanics of respiration during immersion in water', *Journal of Applied Physiology*, 27, 535–8.

Tishler, M. and Y Shoenfeld, 1996, 'Medical and scientific aspects of spa therapy', *Israel Journal of Medical Science*, 32, Sup. 3, 8–10.

The uses of water in spa therapy

3

Thalassotherapy today

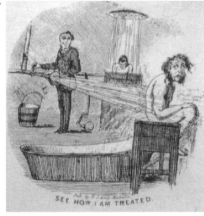

John Winsor Harcup

Cartoon of an early form of Jet blitz or 'douche á jet'

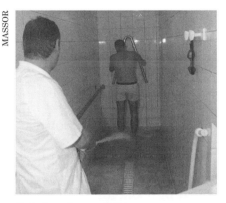

MASSOR

Jet douche or blitz

Modern seawater treatment (thalassotherapy) centres are custom-built, with complex pools of varying depths for different uses; various temperatures of water; horizontal and vertical showers; exercise pools; walking pools; special foot and arm bathing areas; seaweed envelopments and *'douche á jet'* (sometimes called 'blitz') hydromassage machines, which consist of a high-pressure spray of hot seawater followed by a jet of cold seawater to specific areas to achieve circulatory or reflex effects, helping to drain the lymphatic system. The *'douche á jet'* hydromassage treatments all start from the feet and work up to the neck, stimulating each part of the lymphatic system and eventually draining the body of impurities via the urinary tract.

Various mud or sand applications may be used on the joints. Selected muds are very beneficial in both beauty and medical treatments. Mud is said to detoxify, relieve sports strains, arthritis or any area of the body that is swollen, congested or sore. Coastal muds, clay, loam and muds from inland lakes and peat are used for packs. The name given to this group of mud is Peloids (see page 123 Chapter 4) and includes chalk.

As a natural therapy, thermal applications of different kinds of mud were practised in ancient times. The Greek physician, anatomist and physiologist, Galen (129–199 AD), codified the great benefit given by these treatments, particularly in cases of chronic inflammatory diseases, arthritis and rheumatism. Plinius (23–79 AD) mentioned the use of the fango mud from the thermal ponds of Battaglia near Padua in North Italy.

In some centres, small amounts of seawater, containing various trace elements such as magnesium, iodine and other salts may be prescribed for drinking. For example: seawater's potassium content might be used to help fluid retention problems or the fluoride content might be used to help calcium metabolism if this is unbalanced. The water is given undiluted in its natural state or with a fruit juice for palatability. It is not recommended trying this without medical supervision. Drinking seawater is not practised in the UK.

Today, more than 500 000 people a year visit one of the 45 thalassotherapy centres along the 3000 km French coastline. Modern thalassotherapy places an emphasis on treating what the French call *Maladies de la civilisation* – stress, over-tiredness, bad diet, mild depression and pollution. By treating these conditions, it is believed, clients can truly experience wellness – which many people perhaps never experience in their whole life.

The Thermes Marins hotel and thalassotherapy centre in Saint-Malo, France was refurbished in 1963. This coincided with the start of the 'new' thalassotherapy – balancing health – which came to maturity in the 1990s. The Thermes Marins diversified its services by introducing the concept of the 'Aquatonic' labyrinth and devised programmes including hydrotherapy, physiotherapy and seaweed treatments to suit individual needs.

Nowadays you can enjoy a myriad of ultra modern treatments, including **hydro pools** and thalasso pools; thermal mineral pools; **Rasuls**; **Turkish hamman** or **Celtic Roman baths**; **laconium**, caldarium and tropical rain showers. These can help treat arthritis, rheumatism, sports injuries, respiratory or circulatory problem, and obesity, and clients with post-chemotherapy or post-natal conditions.

It is now possible to install pre-formed hydro pools in to almost any location and, by using brine or salt added to tap water, create a 3 per cent mineral salt pool. These pools can be used for relaxation or as part of a monitored physiotherapy or other clinical programme. Hydro pool packs come in various models to create 25sq m pools to cater for 7–8 people, through to 60sq m pools for 26–28 people. A number of high-grade stainless steel water and air attractions can be installed in a variety of pool shapes. Packs usually include airbeds, whirl tubs, neck massage

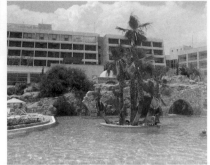

Seawater lagoon, Le Meridien Hotel and Spa, Cyprus

Fascinating Fact

Sea-oil pool
Slightly viscous brown substance with a 47 per cent salt content plus magnesium chloride, that smells of fresh seaweed. Developed by Dr Scarba in Sardinia.

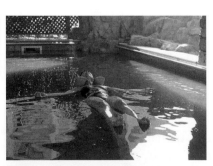

Sea-oil flotation pool, Le Meridien Hotel and Spa, Cyprus

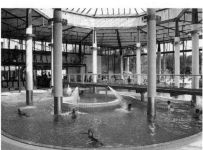

Hydro pool, Terme Radenci, Maribor, Slovenia

fountains, multi-height massage jets, pool rails and all the necessary plant and controls.

Airbeds are constructed of perforated tubes, from which thousands of air bubbles are released. They are equipped with a compressor and are designed to be used as underwater loungers. Thousands of soft air bubbles promote a high level of humidity with a high salt content. This is very relaxing as it creates nearly full body suspension, beneficial for respiratory problems. It also promotes an increase in blood circulation, enabling clients to relax whilst in a reclining, ergonomically correct position.

Whirl tubs or **whirlpools** are activated by a compressor. Thousands of air bubbles massage the feet, legs and entire body; this is especially beneficial for cold feet and heavy legs.

The neck and shoulders are very vulnerable parts of the body and the majority of people will experience stiffness or pain there from time to time, often in relation to stress and pressure. A neck massage fountain is operated by a pump and is designed with a large round, but unpressured, soft water stream to achieve a regular flow. By standing under the fountain, the water flow massages stiff or painful areas on the neck and shoulders. This fountain activates the circulation and relieves aches and pains.

Massage jets can be placed at different heights within the hydro pool walls. Guests can choose the appropriate height of jets to massage the desired part of the body.

In 'purist' terms, a thalassotherapy centre must be less than 500 metres from the coast in a marine climate, using only natural, unpolluted seawater. Pollution can overwhelm the cleansing process and modern thalassotherapy centres require strict testing for contamination. In France industrial complexes, or factories, cannot be built within a 10-kilometre radius of a thalassotherapy centre. The pipelines used to transport the seawater are titanium, ceramic or high-grade stainless steel to avoid contamination and protect against corrosion.

Thalassotherapy centres in France also have to conform to the standards set down by the Fédération de Mer et Santé (sea and health), created in 1986 to guarantee the quality of treatments at the centres, which have to abide by a 'charter of quality'. This imposes strict hygiene standards with the water being drawn from a safe distance and at a depth that will guarantee its purity.

The salt content, radioactivity and bacterial count of the seawater are monitored. In addition, various tests are carried out and precautions taken. Thalassotherapy centres

Fascinating Fact

In 1996, 27 French centres and one Spanish centre agreed to abide by the Quality Charter of the Fédération de Mer et Santé. Centres must:

1. be situated on the coastline
2. use fresh seawater
3. have one or more doctors practising permanently at the centre
4. employ qualified personnel.

in France are under medical or qualified professional supervision with doctors, physiotherapists, kinesiologists, nutritionists and aestheticians, practising from the centre and available at all times.

> **Tip**
>
> Thalassotherapy can be incorporated into an existing Salon or Spa by introducing seaweed envelopment wraps and mud treatments. Also by adding freeze dried sea water or sea mineral salts into a hydrotherapy bath or pool.
>
> These aid biological functions of the body through the absorption of trace elements. Trace elements act as a catalyst to ensure the body functions properly through a proper mineral balance. When we are in a relaxed state our body's functions increase, therefore we are able to absorb the trace elements, vitamins, minerals and enzymes into the body's systems more easily.

Fascinating Fact

An 8-day stay at a thalassotherapy centre is said to restore the balance of the body for 6 months. By having two sessions a year, thalassotherapy can significantly reduce the use of painkillers.

According to the French, thalassotherapy is one of the best ways to mineralise and detoxify the body. When the body is immersed in seawater at a minimum temperature of 33°C for a minimum period of 12 minutes, the absorption of trace elements and minerals by osmosis occurs. This is said to be the equivalent of 20 hours' immersion in the sea at normal climatic temperatures.

The Fédération de Mer et Santé argue that you cannot transport seawater and use it elsewhere. The living organisms of seawater are very fragile. These treatments are designed to have a long-lasting effect, to be of a curative nature, and not just offer short-term relief.

Seawater is used as a means of treating a wide range of ailments and also good for keeping the body fit. The salt content in the world's oceans, which is thought to account

Table 3.1 Mineral content of Red Sea and Mediterranean Sea (grams per litre)

	$NaCl$	$MgCl_2$	$CaCl_2$	KCl	$MgBr_2$	$CaSo_4$	$MgSo_4$	Total grams/ litre
Dead Sea	86 (29%)	132 (41%)	35 (12%)	11 (4%)	9 (3%)	7 (2%)	20 (14%)	300
Mediterranean Sea	27 (77%)	4 (11%)	(0.3%)	(0.3%)	(0.3%)	2 (3%)	2 (6%)	35

for the benefits of thalassotherapy, is around 35 grams per litre, rising to 42 grams per litre in the Red Sea, and higher still in the Dead Sea, where the salinity is up to 10 times that of an open ocean. The Dead Sea is known as the Salt Sea, due to this extremely high concentration of salts and minerals. Table 3.1 compares the mineral content of the Dead Sea and the Mediterranean Sea.

Climatotherapy

A variation of thalassotherapy is climatotherapy, which involves the use of unique qualities of the air and climate. Traditionally, aerosols using seawater for inhalation were used to help respiratory problems and smokers; some countries now use sterile saline.

The prevailing sea breezes, which carry sea spray, become charged with particles of salt water and iodine in suspension. The fields of seaweed, uncovered at low tide, perfume the air and are carried by the winds coming straight from the sea, free from any dust and pollution. This fresh air, loaded with sea spray relieves congestion and clears the breathing passages. Sea air contains a large proportion of negative *ions* and is rich in iodine (which helps to regulate the metabolism). Sea air is also relatively pure; in the centre of a large city, one cubic metre of air contains 50 000 microbes, this drops to 150 per cubic metre in unpolluted coastal areas.

According to the Fédération de Mer et Santé, each coastal climate is a remedy in its own way – the English Channel coast is *vivifiant* (stimulating), the Atlantic coast is

Fascinating Fact

Our moods can be affected by *ions* in the atmosphere. These are electrically charged atoms or groups of atoms, having a negative or positive charge, depending on whether they have gained or lost an electron. Positive ions build up in certain circumstances – prior to a thunder storm for instance – and can result in headaches, depression, irritability, lethargy and a general feeling of malaise. In contrast, the preponderance of negative ions after a storm brings relief from tension, headaches and the return of energy and happiness. Many familiar things in modern day living destroy negative ions including pollution, air-conditioning, central heating, dust, electrical appliances and synthetic fibres.

Fascinating Fact

Some spas have 'ionising rooms' (cavitosonic rooms) to combat a build-up of positive ions. Ionisers for the home are available from chemists and health food shops and can help those with breathing problems.

Moving water, mountain streams and waves breaking on the shore all produce negative ions which augment our feel-good factor when we are near them.

Therefore, moving water as in airbeds, hydrobaths, neck fountains, mists, showers and whirlpools are all part of the spa scene, creating an oasis of negative ions in our modern urban world.

tonique (invigorating) and the Mediterranean is *sédatif* (calming). The physiological and pathological effects of a specific climate on the human body take into account the following factors:

- temperature/altitude/latitude
- humidity
- air purity/microbes
- sunshine/radiation
- light
- winds
- ecology/flora and fauna
- location of sea/large surfaces of water/mountains/ glaciers.

The effects of light on the body are due to action on the cells of the body and antagonistic action on parasitic microbes. Sunlight has an antiseptic action on exposed microbes. The sea and sun (NSUP – natural selective ultraviolet photo therapy) provide the basis of treatment for different skin and joint diseases, especially psoriasis, though patients with atopic dermatitis, vitiligo, ichtiosis and acne also respond well to this treatment.

Because of the unique location of the Dead Sea, certain atmospheric, thermal and chemical characteristics are found there that do not exist anywhere else in the world. The Dead Sea is located 400 metres below sea level (it is the lowest place on earth); it is 80 km long and 17 km wide. The Sea has two basins: one in the north, 350 metres deep, and the other in the south, a shallow pool just a few metres deep.

The Dead Sea is situated between mountains that rise to 1200m, with over 300 days of sunshine per year and temperatures in the range of 22–29°C from November to April, up to 39°C in July. The temperature is rarely below +10°C. The average atmospheric pressure is about 1050–1066 millibars. The oxygen content in the air is 10 per cent higher than at the sea level.

There is a heavy haze over the Dead Sea at all times due to extremely high evaporation (about 2 billion m³ per year). This haze and the additional 400 metres of atmosphere help to filter out more UVB rays (which can cause sunburn), and create the ideal correlation of UVA and UVB rays, so that the duration of exposure to the sun can be increased.

These geographical characteristics combine to provide a treatment known as bioclimatology. Bioclimatology is used for certain diseases of the skin: psoriasis, atopic dermatitis and vitiligo. Arthritis and other types of rheumatic dysfunction also respond extremely well to this type of treatment. Highly trained dermatologists and rheumatologists practise in clinics offering personalised programmes, which greatly improve these skin conditions.

Other aspects of climate

Ozone, an allotropic form of oxygen, has a disinfectant action and is augmented by intense sunlight. Apparently ozone is increased during storms and is more abundant in spring and autumn. Less ozone is found in houses and towns than in the open country.

Dry air is more bracing than moist air. It is easier to work or live in a dry climate than one with high humidity. Moist air combined with cold can aggravate catarrh and rheumatic conditions. Understanding pollution, pollen, dust and other factors at work in the atmosphere can enable the spa practitioner to utilise different prevailing climatic conditions to treat a range of problems.

Exercise in water

Therapeutic effects of exercise in water

Exercising in water can be traced back to the training of Roman centurions and soldiers. This form of exercise increases muscle power and endurance and helps to mobilise joints and muscles. With the buoyancy and support of water, it is the perfect medium for helping muscles to relax and improving co-ordination.

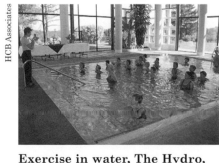

The buoyancy of water reduces the body's weight by up to 90 per cent. Expectant mothers are one group who can exercise effortlessly in water without putting any strain on themselves or their baby. Exercises can be done with a partner, either working together or offering support. Government reports state that 30 minutes of physical activity will greatly improve the body's health and well-being by aiding weight reduction and reducing the risk of heart disease and osteoporosis.

Exercise in water, The Hydro, Stellanbosch, South Africa

The benefits of exercising in water are that it:

- stretches and strengthens muscles, increasing flexibility and muscular release by relaxation
- increases a range of movement
- helps to develop muscles
- soothes painful joints and frees movements in arthritic conditions
- aids balance, co-ordination, agility and neuromuscular facilitation
- improves spinal alignment and balance with gentle bodywork
- aids recovery from injury, stroke and especially in sports injury musculoskeletal operations
- improves breathing pattern
- increases oxygen consumption
- may lower blood pressure levels
- helps reduce or prevent obesity (in conjunction with dietary restraint)
- helps multiple sclerosis sufferers to improve their mobility
- calms the mind and reduces stress and anxiety
- improves insomnia
- increases metabolism and blood circulation.

Aquatic agility

The following are typical exercise movements in water (each movement is usually performed three times):

- head flexion and extension
- shoulder circles back and forth
- arm swinging back and forth
- leg swinging back and forth
- arm flexion and extension
- straight arm swinging back and forth
- small and big steps in place
- leg flexion and extension
- head circles
- arm side swings
- shoulder up and down
- leg swinging to the side, leg circles
- arm circles
- head side bends
- trunk side.

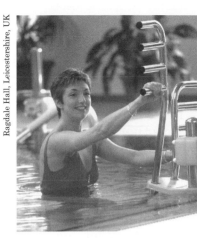

Exercise with equipment in water, Ragdale Hall, Leicestershire, UK

PEPs – Pool Exercise Programmes

In co-operation with the Arthritis Foundation, Pool Exercise Programmes have been developed to increase and maintain joint flexibility, to strengthen and tone muscles and as an exercise plan to maintain healthy joints. There are two programmes:

1. *Basic* – 11 series of exercises with 42 gentle movements, designed to exercise a specific joint or muscle group. Using a range of slow motion, strengthening and endurance exercises to help maintain normal joint movement, relieve stiffness or restore flexibility. The basic programme commences with a warm-up, with the body part-submerged in water, followed by strengthening and endurance exercises and finishes with a cool down to prevent blood from pooling in the muscles.

2. *Plus* – 7 activities in addition to the basic programme. A series of combined arm and leg movements, performed at a faster and more continuous pace.

Source: MSA, PO Box 282, Fawnskin, CA 9233-0282 USA.

The Shaw method

This was created and developed by Steven Shaw and his wife Limor, this method is based on the principles of the **Alexander Technique** and allows the body to swim without putting any stress on the neck, back and knees.

Balneotherapy

Balneotherapy and balneology are both derived from the Latin, balneum, meaning bath. Balneotherapy means the treatment of disease by baths. Balneology is the scientific study of using bathing in medicine. Some authors consider balneotherapy to be a subdivision of hydrotherapy. Strictly speaking this is correct as hydrotherapy, a word coined in 1876 is derived from hydro meaning water, and literally means water treatment. It embraces all kinds of bathing – thermal and cold baths, mineral and hydrobaths and whirlpools.

Hydrotherapy techniques also use sitz baths, baths at different temperatures (contrast baths), vapour baths, baths for limbs, **Vichy** or **affusion showers** and the Scottish douche. All these relate to spa therapy. Hydrotherapy can mean 'any therapeutic use of water'.

In 1843, the term hydrotherapy was preceded by hydropathy, which specifically meant the internal and external application of water in the treatment of disease as in the Water Cure discussed in Chapter 1.

Balneotherapy includes some aspects of hydrotherapy, in addition to other forms of bathing – for example mud, peat, and algae wraps. In simple terms, balneotherapy is the use of bathing whether in a hydrotherapy bath or pool. Balneotherapy treatments can have different purposes. In a spa setting, they can be used to treat conditions such as arthritis and backache, build up muscles after injury or illness or to stimulate the immune system, and they can be enjoyed as a relief from day-to-day stress – or even just for fun.

One of the positive effects of water on the body is a sense of well-being. Balneotherapy/hydrotherapy is recognised by the medical profession as a part of physiotherapy. Exercises in water are carried out by physiotherapists specially trained for rehabilitation treatment. Water treatments are used therapeutically for the physical and psychological care of a wide variety of conditions. The psychological effects of water and its ability to relieve day-to-day stress should never be underestimated.

Some of the therapeutic effects of warm bathing are:

1. *De-stress* – A warm bath relaxes the body, soothes tight muscles and sore areas. It provides a sense of well-being and relaxation.

2. *Increases blood circulation in the skin* – This aids the removal of the dead tissue layer on the surface of the skin, which in turn increases cellular renewal. The skin is nourished by the absorption of small amounts of minerals, vitamins, trace elements and amino acids.

3. *Aids biological function* – Warm bathing helps the absorption of trace elements which act as a catalyst to ensure the body functions properly by having a proper mineral balance.

Fascinating Fact

Specially trained hydrotherapists now treat post-operative, post-injury, neurological conditions, strokes, brain damage, and Parkinson's disease. These techniques are being used in a small number of pools run by the NHS (National Health Service, UK) and privately.

Effects of hydro massage

The physiological effects of massage with water should not be underestimated. They often contribute to making a client feel healthier, invigorated and more energetic.

Underwater massage (**hydro massage**) can be used to increase pressure and muscular stimulation without

Fascinating Fact

'Health is not just the absence of disease but the total state of well being – physical, mental and spiritual' (World Health Organisation definition of good health).

placing any effort or stress on the heart. It can allow the body to eliminate toxins, through perspiration, muscular stimulation and lymphatic drainage.

Many people suffer from stress. They find that hydrotherapy promotes relaxation as it soothes away minor aggravating aches and pains. Some clients feel that regular hydrotherapy keeps them looking younger, and because of improvements in their skin they are encouraged to pay more attention to proper nutrition, exercise and healthy living.

Benefits and effects of balneotherapy/hydrotherapy, including exercise in water

*Improves the **circulatory system** by:*
Altering heart action to develop a stronger heart
Increasing circulation
Increasing oxygen supply to cells
Increasing the supply of nutrients to cells
Removing metabolic waste
Decreasing swelling of the limbs
(May decrease high blood pressure)

*Improves the **digestive system** by:*
Relaxing the abdominal and intestinal muscles
Relieving anxiety (which adversely affects digestion)
Stimulating the activity of the liver
Removal of waste material

*Improves the **metabolic system** by:*
Altering the metabolic rate
Reducing obesity – when combined with proper diet and exercise

*Improves the **renal system** by:*
Increasing kidney function
Stimulating the elimination of water and waste products

*Improves the **muscular system** by:*
Relaxing muscles
Stimulating and strengthening muscles
Relieving pain, tension and stiffness – especially pain in the shoulders, neck and back, often caused by strain and poor posture

*Improves the **nervous system** by:*
Stimulating sensory nerves
Relieving restlessness, stress and insomnia
Suppression of the sympathetic nervous system

*Improves the **respiratory system** by:*
Exercising and stimulating respiratory muscles
Re-educating normal breathing patterns

*Improves the **lymphatic system** by:*
Stimulating lymphatic drainage in all areas of the body

*Improves the **immune system** by:*
Stimulating T-Cell lymphocytes and other white cells
Acting as if the body had been challenged by an infective agent, such as a bacterium or virus

*Improves the **skin** by:*
Stimulating the cutaneous circulation to improve tone, elasticity, colour and texture
Improving the nutrition of skin cells
Encouraging absorption of trace elements into skin cells

*Improves the **skeletal system** by:*
Increasing the flexibility of joints
Removing excess fluid from joints
Exercising to realign correct posture
Encouraging better balance reactions

__Psychological__ changes
Relaxes the mind as well as the body
Induces a sense of well-being and euphoria
Mental and physical fatigue is diminished and energy is promoted

Advanced water therapies

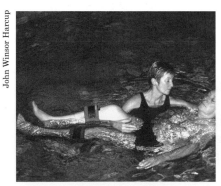

John Winsor Harcup

Watsu, The Bath House, The Royal Crescent Hotel and Spa, Bath, UK

Many water therapies have developed combining the knowledge of ancient oriental therapies and aquatic bodywork to provide relaxation at a deeper level, freedom of movement, spirituality and to unblock the energy channels and restore the chi or energy.

Watsu

Watsu evolved in 1980 as the first form of aquatic bodywork when Harold Dull was floating his **Zen shiatsu** students in a warm pool at Harbin Hot Springs, California. The name is derived from the two words WAter and shiaTSU. It is considered to be the most profound development of aquatic shiatsu bodywork allowing a greater freedom of movement, encouraging trust through connection and touch by freeing the body in water.

It is performed by lying back supported in the warm water; being allowed to sink and rise to the rhythm of your breathing, leading to a feeling of weightlessness and being nurtured in the water, thus releasing emotions. When the body is continually moving in the water and each movement is flowing into the next, the mind cannot anticipate what is going to happen. There is no resistance and the body can move freely without pain and go into positions that it would be impossible if fear were present.

Some of the benefits of Watsu are that it:

- stretches and strengthens muscles, increasing flexibility
- increases a range of motion
- improves breathing patterns
- improves insomnia and reduces stress and anxiety.

It is important that the water is warm and does not exceed 37°C (98°F). The Watsu practitioner should familiarise themselves with the client and ascertain any precautions, or contra-indications:

- movements that might be worsened by pressure or movement e.g. arching the back.
- neck or back problems – avoid movements that are uncomfortable
- muscle tension
- disc problems – may become aggravated
- varicose veins – avoid pressing on them
- areas of inflammation i.e. sprains or tendonitis – avoid pressure or excessive movements on them
- phlebitis
- the elderly – use gentle movements with them in case they have brittle bones
- persons who have a condition that does not allow long periods of time to be spent in the water.

Trust, fear and limitations are extremely important for the Watsu practitioner to understand almost on an intuitive level, as there is a closeness or intimacy with Watsu. It is important that Watsu is performed with slow movements to avoid the client feeling dizzy or nauseous.

Learning to breathe correctly, sink and float are all part of the Watsu experience. There are other disciplines that can be done on land to make the body more supple and the mind more centred, for example tai chi, **meditation** and yoga.

The nose and ears should be kept out of the water, but nose pegs can be worn. Some people have a tendency to ear infections or are bothered by the water entering the ear, and again ear plugs can be worn.

Water dance

'Wassertanzen' (Wa Ta) is a form of aquatic bodywork created in Germany by Arjana Brunschwiler and Aman Schroter in 1987. It is similar to Watsu as the guest is cradled, stretched and relaxed in water. In Wa Ta, the whole body is taken below the water with the aid of nose clips and is thus freed from the bounds of gravity. The body is then moved and stretched, incorporating the massage elements of Aikido, dolphin and snake movements with rolls, dance and somersaults. This can induce a physical release of emotions and a deep state of relaxation.

Hydroholistics

Developed by Hilary Austin, a Watsu/Wa Ta practitioner and an Alexander Technique teacher, hydroholistics combines Watsu and Alexander Technique principles. This technique provides freedom for the body in water with Watsu, which is followed by a session on land that encourages ease of movement using Alexander Techniques in relation to posture.

Jahara

The Jahara technique, developed by Mario Jahara, in Ohai, California is based on an understanding of the physiology of the body and the physical properties of water. It develops skills that allow the person to work one-on-one, under and above the water, in a stress-free environment. This technique works without the need for effort or physical strength, by allowing the client to float in water, integrating freedom using support and skills with a sound understanding of the principles and practice of the movements involved.

There are three principles:

1. *Jahara Basics* – learning to float people safely, comfortably and creatively in water, providing body support and aquatic bodywork.

2. *Jahara Expansion* – the emphasis of this principle is on spinal alignment with gentle bodywork and muscular release by expansion. Adaptability and creativity are required to achieve this technique.

3. *Jahara Underwater* – the focus at this stage is on a continuous flowing movement, using breath control under and above the water.

Ai Chi

Read treatment card 'Use and Application of Ai Chi'.

Ai Chi is a water exercise and relaxation method combining deep breathing and slow movement, using a blend of Eastern and Western methods of tai chi, shiatsu, Watsu and aquatic exercise.

The benefits of Ai Chi are:

- improved mobility and agility
- increased metabolism and blood circulation
- increased energy consumption
- increased oxygen consumption by 7 per cent
- improved liver efficiency
- improved balance, co-ordination, symmetry and neuromuscular facilitation
- a calm mind – decreased stress
- relief of joint and muscular pain.

When practising Ai Chi, the pool should be shoulder deep – 1.3 metres – with a temperature of 35°C in a calm

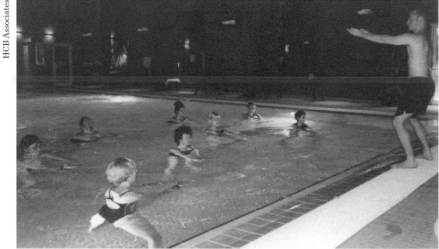

HCB Associates

A class of Ai Chi performed at Nirvana Spa, Sindlesham, UK

The Use and Application of Ai Chi

Benefit of treatment

Ai Chi uses a combination of Eastern and Western methods of Tai Chi, Shiatsu, Watsu and aquatic exercise that will increase the metabolism and blood circulation, increase oxygen consumption by 7%, improve liver efficiency as well as balance, co-ordination, symmetry and neuromuscular facilitation.

Advantages

Ai Chi helps those with problems of balance, movement and agility. Relieves joint and muscular pain and decreases stress and insomnia.

Contra-indications

- Low Blood pressure
- Skin diseases, such as severe eczema or open psoriasis
- Uncontrolled epilepsy
- Heavy periods

Preparation

When practising Ai Chi, the pool depth should be shoulder depth – 1.3 meters with a temperature of 35°c in a calm environment
Make sure that your shoulders are under the water, knees slightly bent and body relaxed.

Method

BREATHING MOVEMENT – Repeat each movement 3–5 times:

- **Stationary**
  Place hands in front of you, palms facing down and breathe gently as you exhale through the mouth, lower the arms 12cms keeping them straight at the same time. As you inhale through the nose, turn wrist so palms face upwards and raise arms to just below the surface of the water.

- **Front raise**
  Hold arms horizontal, in front of you, palms facing down. Lower arms to the thigh, keeping them straight, at the same time, slowly exhale through the mouth. Turn wrists so palms face forward, raise arms, keeping them straight and slowly inhale through the nose.

- **Side raise**
  From a vertical arm position, palms facing forward, raise arms to the side, keeping them straight and at the same time, inhale through the nose. As you reach the surface turn wrists so palms face down and slowly exhale through the mouth lowering arms back to vertical position.

- **Horizontal side to front**
  From horizontal position, palms face up, turn wrists so palms face down, bring arms to the

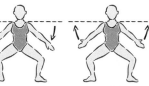

front, keeping them straight and exhale through the mouth, until the hands meet. Turn palms to face up and return arm position to the side, keeping them straight and inhale through the nose, stretching back as far as possible to expand the chest cavity.

- **Front centre cross**
  From side horizontal position, palms facing up, turn palms to face down, lower arms and gradually cross to the front of your body, exhale through the mouth, turn palms to face up, keeping elbows close to the body, uncross arms to expand chest cavity and exhale through the nose.

UPPER BODY MOVEMENTS   Turn body and repeat each movement to the other side

- **Front half swing**
  From side horizontal position, palms facing down, swing right arm over to the left arm, keeping face forward, exhale through the mouth until contact then turn right wrist, palm facing up, return arm to horizontal side position, inhale through the nose.

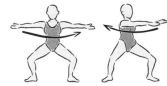

- **Rear half swing**
  From side horizontal position, palms facing down, take right arm over to the left turning body and exhale through the mouth.
  Turn left wrist, palms facing up, swing your left arm behind you, keeping face and right arm forward, inhale through the nose. Turn left wrist, palm facing down and return to your right arm and exhale through your mouth.
  Repeat 3–5 times. Turn right wrist, palm facing up, swing right arm over to the right to return to starting position, inhale through the nose.

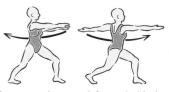

- **Full turn swing**

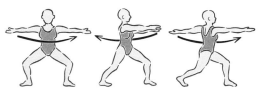

This movement is the same as the rear half swing, but it is all one movement – 360° turn.
From side horizontal position, palms facing down, swing right arm and body to the left, exhale through the mouth. Turn left wrist, palms facing up and swing arm back as far as possible whilst following your hand with your head, inhale through your nose.
Return to centre position and repeat on the other side.

After care

- Shower
- Drink plenty of still water
- Relax

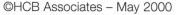

www.spa-therapy.com   ©HCB Associates – May 2000

environment. Make sure that your shoulders are under the water, knees slightly bent and body relaxed. Perform the exercise with slow, large movements using the whole body. Turn the palms of your hands upward when inhaling and turn your palms downward when exhaling.

Ai Chi can be performed in pairs and this is called Ai Chi Ne. See 'The Use and Application of Ai Chi' step-by-step guide opposite.

Dreams and rituals in healing water

The powers of dreams, imagination and creativity are explored during this treatment. A sequence of activities and times are spent floating in different states of consciousness. This procedure is based on ancient Egyptian and Greek healing methods of sound and water, where a deeply personal and visionary discovery into the language of dreams is encountered.

Liquid Sound

During a **Liquid Sound** treatment, light and music are used under and above the water for a relaxation and visualisation that revolutionises the conventional bathing experience. The body and soul are in complete harmony whilst bathed in sound, colour and light. You feel the vibrations of music on your body – in the water.

> *Sheltered and secure as an embryo in the womb, you emerge as if reborn.*
>
> *(Micky Remann, Liquid Sound)*

Aqua Wellness

Aqua Wellness is a combination of gentle stretching movements, **deep tissue massage** and joint release that will rock, sway and swing the body effortlessly in warm water. This aqua bodywork benefits the radius of the joint, as the movements allow the whole spine to swing weightlessly in the healing energies of the warm water.

A session of Aqua Wellness commences with a relaxation phase on the surface of the water. When the body and mind are in a deeply relaxed state, the second phase of taking the body underwater begins, and the body is gently submerged. The Aqua Wellness 'Bodyworker' will work along with the client, monitoring the rhythms of breathing.

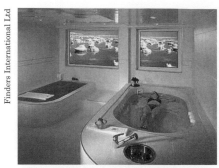

Flotation pool and room by Finders International, Kent, UK

Finders International Ltd

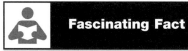

Fascinating Fact

Lilly was the first neuroscientist to map the brain of a chimpanzee and he is the inventor of the 'Lilly Wave', an electrical pulse that can stimulate the brain while not damaging it.

Fascinating Fact

Epsom Salts is the common name for magnesium sulphate, made of a similar composition to the salts found at the wells in Epsom, Surrey, UK, known to have a purgative effect. They can be taken as a drink, used in the bath, or used as a topical application.

Tip

REST:
Restricted
Environment
Stimulation
Therapy
– sound and light deprivation to minimalise normal brain stimuli.

Flotation

Flotation therapy can be experienced in salt and mineral rich seas, natural lakes and brine baths (e.g. the Dead Sea in the Middle East and the brine baths at Droitwich in the UK) or in pools and tanks. Research (Randolfi 1997 and Lilly 1958) has shown that sensory deprivation – lack of light, sound and gravity, combined with the body floating in water at a thermoneutral temperature – induces deep relaxation – a meditative state, known as the *Theta* state, which is the optimum period for cells of the body to reproduce and rejuvenate in a healthy environment.

Dr John C. Lilly, an American neuro-physiologist and psychoanalyst famous for his work with relationships between human beings and dolphins, investigated sensory deprivation. He assumed that by creating a deep state of relaxation, the brain would sleep or switch off. He discovered that the brain when freed of physical stimulation (this accounts for 90 per cent of normal brain activity) and in a deep relaxing state, opens the mind to imagination, creativity and problem solving – compare this to a computer de-fragmenting.

In 1954, Lilly developed the sensory isolation **flotation tank**, using a solution of Epsom Salts in an enclosed shallow pool to create a buoyancy similar to that of the Dead Sea. Lilly reviewed his research on the brain and mind and human consciousness using this tank.

The physical benefits of flotation therapy are numerous. However, further research is required to establish the therapeutic benefits for both physical and mental health in the case of chronic conditions, post-operative care, disability, rehabilitation or sports injuries. The physical benefits include:

- muscle tension is reduced
- veins and capillaries dilate
- oxygen and nutrients are transported to cells more efficiently
- the pulse rate is lowered
- adrenaline (epinephine) and cortisol levels are lowered, reducing stress
- endorphins are released, relieving pain
- breathing rate is lowered.

It is recommended that a session of two hours is required to appreciate the full effects of flotation, however, the usual 20–40 minute sessions are long enough to experience the benefits. Some clients find a tank or capsule claustrophobic and there are now companies developing open pools. These are becoming more popular as they allow the client to move about more freely.

Contra-indications

There are a number of contra-indications and precautions to be observed when undertaking water therapies and aquatic exercises where the body is in water for long periods of time, such as Ai Chi, Watsu, Wa Ta and Liquid Sound, etc.

- *Severe urinary tract infection* with frequency of micturition (urination) and/or feelings of urgency, because of the possibility of involuntary release of urine into the water.
- *Patients with a catheter* can use pools provided the bag or bladder is drained.
- *Unpredictable bowel incontinence and diarrhoea (within 48 hours)* – risk of pool pollution and the release of E-coli bacilli and organic matter which overloads the disinfectant system.
- *Open wounds* – excess immersion delays healing.
- *Skin disease* – severe eczema/psoriasis with cracked skin or infection.
- *Contagious water or air-borne infection* – e.g. legionella and various virus infections.
- *Epilepsy, if uncontrolled by drugs* – light reflecting off the water may stimulate abnormal brain activity.
- *Absence of cough reflex* – as after stroke or brain injury, because of the increased risk of drowning.
- *Sensitivity to pool chemicals*, such as bromine, rarely chlorine.
- *Recent cerebral haemorrhage* – wait 3 weeks and seek supervised rehabilitation.
- *Impaired skin sensation* – through stroke, brain injury, spinal cord injury, diabetic neuropathy, severe peripheral arterial disease and other causes.
- *Perforated ear drums* – unless water is kept out of the ears with ear plugs.
- *Severe kidney disease* – where patient cannot adjust to fluid loss.
- *Patient with impaired ability to regulate body temperature* as a result of brain damage.
- *Gastrostomies/colostomies/iliostomies* – can enter the pool if stoma is well healed and the bag is securely fixed and has been drained.

- *Heat sensitivity* – some underwater lights can generate considerable heat – do not allow clients to lean against them.
- *Multiple sclerosis* – may be extra sensitive to heat.
- *After radiation therapy and long-term steroids*, especially topical steroids, the skin is thin and extra sensitive.

References

Abels, D.J., Theodore, M.D. and Jacob E.Bearman, 1995, 'Treatment of psoriasis at a Dead Sea Mor Dermatology clinic', *International Journal of Dermatology*, 34/2.

Abels, Kattan-Byron J. 1985, 'Psoriasis treatment at the Dead Sea', *Journal of the American Academy of Dermatology*, 12, 639–43.

Committee on Guidelines of Care, Task Force on Phototherapy and Photo Chemotherapy, 1994, 'Guidelines of care for phototherapy and photo chemotherapy', *Journal of the American Academy of Dermatology*, 31, 643–8.

Dull, Harold, 1997, *WATSU Freeing the Body in Water*, 2nd edn, Harbin Springs Publishing.

Gold, B., S. Sukenic, and Z. Gavza, 1990, 'Radioactivity and chemical composition of the therapeutic mud and hot spring baths in the Moriah Spa, Dead Sea, Israel', in E. Riklis (ed.), *Frontiers in Radiation Biology*, Balabak, 625–30.

Gumon, Even-Paz R., V. Kipnis, D. Abels and D. Efron, 1994, 'Dead Sea sun *Versus* Dead Sea water in the treatment of psoriasis', paper given at Mediterranean Conference Center, Malta, November.

Kipnis, V. 1995, Dead Sea Mor Dermatology Clinic, Israel.

Kushelevsky, A.P., 1988, 'A review of some important biometeorological factors at the Dead Sea', *Journal of Medical Science*, Department of Nuclear Engineering Ben Gurion University, Israel.

Lobban, Christopher S. and Paul J. Harrison. 1997, *Seaweed Ecology and Physiology*, Cambridge University Press, Cambridge.

Ryrie, Charlie, 1998, *The Healing Energies of Water*, Gaia Books, London.

Weber, Sir Hermann and F. Parkes Weber, 1907, *Climatotherapy and Balneotherapy, Health Resorts (Spas) of Europe and North Africa*, Smith, Elder & Co., London.

Useful addresses

Aquatonic Labyrinth, Hotel Thermes Marin, St. Malo, Brittany, France.

Hilary Austin, Hydroholistics, email: hydrohilary@yahoo.com

Fédération International de Thalassothérapie Mer et Sante 8, rue de l'Isly, 75008 Paris, France.

Finders International, Kent, TN17 2JY, UK. www.findershealth.com

Floatworld Limited, email: info@floatworld.com

Sally Hill, specialist in hydrotherapy and flotation, therapeutic and rehabilitation water treatments, email: sallyhill@talk21.com

Institute for Aqua-Wellness – Wunderwaldstr. 2* D-99518, Bad Sulza, Germany. Email: water4view@aol.com, www.liquid-sound.com, www.aquawellness.com

ISA – International Seaweed Association, www.intseaweedassoc.org.

Maison de la France, 178 Piccadilly, London W1J 9AL.

PEP. MSA. PO Box 282, Fawnskin, CA 9233-0282 USA.

WABA (Worldwide Aquatic Bodywork Association), an educational non-profit organisation. P.O.Box 889, Middletown, CA 95461 USA. Email: info@waba.edu

(Seaweed pictures from the Seaweed Site©1995–2002 Michael D. Guiry.)

Therapies in spas

4

Treatments and procedures

In this chapter we will be reviewing therapies for a spa, describing spa treatments, their benefits, precautions and contra-indications. We shall be dealing with the safety, hygiene and maintenance necessary to make the operations of the spa safe and successful.

The core therapies are the most essential part, or innermost part, of the spa. They provide the basis on which to develop more sophisticated therapies. We also describe more sophisticated and advanced therapies that are either popular in spas today or, in our opinion, are likely to become so.

We have included 'step-by-step' treatment procedures for spa treatments. These provide all the essential detail necessary for the most effective use and operation of spa equipment. These informative treatment guides provide an important reference to enable you to operate equipment efficiently and effectively and to carry out treatments. The treatment cards can be downloaded from the website www.spa-therapy.com and then laminated as a practical reference guide, which can be used in a wet environment.

Water is an essential element of spa. The International Spa Association's Ten Domains of the Spa Experience, list water as the first domain as the heart of the spa experience. The full list of ten domains is:

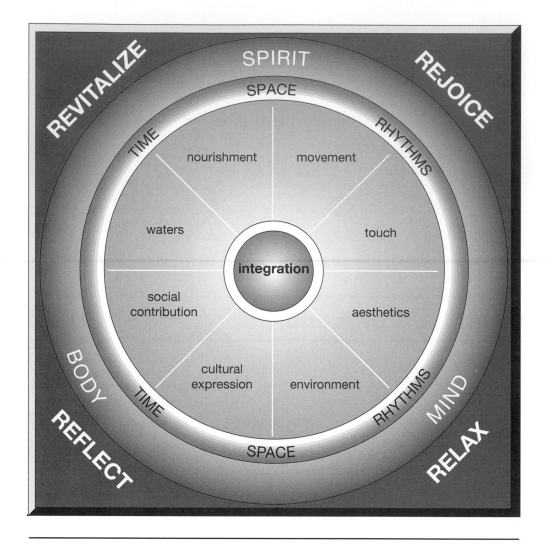

1. Waters: The internal and external use of water in its many forms.

2. Nourishment: What we feed ourselves: food, herbals, supplements, and medicines.

3. Movement: Vitality and energy through movement, exercise, stretching and fitness.

4. Touch: Connectivity and communication embraced through touch, massage and bodywork.

5. Integration: The personal and social relationship between mind, body, spirit and environment.

6. Aesthetics: Our concept of beauty and how botanical agents relate to the biochemical components of the body.

7. Environment: Location, placement, weather patterns, water constitution, natural agents and social responsibility.

8. Cultural Expression: The spiritual belief systems, the value of art and the scientific and political view of the time.

9. Social Contribution: Commerce, volunteer efforts, and intention as they relate to well-being.

10. Time, Space Rhythms: The perception of space and time and its relationship to natural cycles and rhythms.

Circle concept created by R. Zill for ISPA 2001

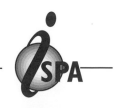

ISPA would like to thank the ISPA education committees past and present.

ISPA wheel created by Robin Zill, President, Touch America Inc. Hillsborough, N. Carolina, USA

Core therapies

The core therapies can be divided into five groups.

1. **Hot:** The sensation caused in the body as a result of different temperatures

    - **sauna** (Tyrolean/laconium/Finnish)
    - steam (caldarium/hamman/cabinet/Roman)
    - aromatic herbal bath
    - Dry Float (Soft Pack)
    - Rasul (Serail)
    - Japanese salt bath

2. **Cold:** The use of very cold or frozen products to vaso-constrict the skin and muscle and create a lift in the skin.

    - **cryotherapy**
    - ice fountain
    - ice room (frigidarium)

3. **Water:** Our life is dependent on water. In the spa it is used in treatments whether thermal water, seawater, sweet water or simply for drinking. The term hydrotherapy can mean 'any therapeutic use of water'. Hydrotherapy treatments can have different purposes. In a spa setting, it can be used to treat conditions such as arthritis and backache, build up muscles after injury or illness or to stimulate the immune system, and it can be enjoyed as a relief from day-to-day stress and for fun (see Chapter 3 'The Uses of Water in Spa Therapy')

    - hydrotherapy (bath/pool/tub)
    - flotation
    - pool
    - hydro shower
    - jet blitz (douche a Jet/Scottish douche)
    - experience shower
    - affusion shower (Vichy)
    - jacuzzi
    - aqua meditation
    - Ai Chi
    - Liquid Sound
    - Kneipp therapy
    - Watsu
    - pedidarium (reflexology basins)

4. **Touch:** The experience or feeling of hands, texture or the quality of objects when they come into contact with the body.

- massage
- envelopment treatments
- cody salt/soap scrubs
- chakra therapy table

5. **Relaxation:** A wide range of methods that will help relax both the mind and body.

- tepidarium
- meditation
- sound therapy
- colour therapy
- Zen garden

Note: *Exercise*, which must be considered a core therapy in spas, should be considered the sixth core element, but is too big a subject to be dealt with in this book.

The treatments offered in a spa treat the five senses:

1. sight
2. sound
3. smell
4. touch
5. taste.

The mind receives information about the external world or the state of the body (happiness, pain, temperature, relaxation, etc.) through these five senses. The addition of spa products to the treatments not only enhances the therapy but also stimulates the five senses. Across the world there is an abundance of natural plants, organic material or local hand-crafted items that can be used, with imagination, to therapeutically or decoratively create spa treatments.

Pre-treatments

Exfoliation

Exfoliation is the removal of dead skin cells by products, loofah rub or body brush.

Body scrub

Body scrub is the exfoliation of dead skin cells using various combinations of sea salt, essential oils, water, skin brush or **loofah** to massage the body and leave the skin feeling silky soft.

Brossage

Brossage is a fine body polish using salicylic salt and brushes, that literally leaves the skin glowing, soft and silky.

Brush and tone

Brush and tone is a stimulating body exfoliating treatment, using skin brushes to dry brush the skin to remove dead layers and impurities whilst stimulating the circulation. Used as a pre-treatment for mud and seaweed body masks. A moisturising lotion completes the treatment, leaving the skin silky smooth.

Salt glow

A **salt glow** is a hydrating and exfoliating treatment consisting of salt, essential oils and water that are massaged over the body to eliminate dead skin cells, leaving the skin very soft and fragrant. This is followed by a shower and application of body lotion to complete the treatment.

Dulse scrub

A **dulse scrub** is an exfoliating body scrub with a mixture of dulse seaweed (sometimes in powder form), oil and water to deep-cleanse and re-mineralize the skin. The skin is gently massaged, leaving the skin incredibly smooth. This is a very relaxing treatment and one that is generally practised in Sweden and Ireland.

Heat treatments

1. Sauna
   - Finnish
     Read treatment card on page 73 'The Use and Application of the Thermarium Sauna and Saunarium'

- Tyrolean
  Read treatment card on page 74, 'The Use and
  Application of the Tyrolean Sauna'
- Laconium
  Read treatment card on page 75, 'The Use and
  Application of the Laconium'

2. Steam

- Caldarium
  Read treatment card on page 76, 'The Use and
  Application of the Caldarium'
- Hamman
  Read treatment card on page 77, 'The Use and
  Application of the Turkish Hamman'
- Thalatherm
  Read treatment card on page 78, The 'Use and
  Application of the Thalatherm'

3. Adaptations of heat treatments

- Aromatic (Greek) herbal bath
  Read treatment card on page 79, 'The Use and
  Application of the Aromatic Herb Bath'
- Dry Flotation on page 81, 'The Use and Application of
  the Dry Float Soft Pack System'
- Rasul
- Serail
- Japanese salt bath
- Kraxen stove®
- **Japanese enzyme bath** (cedar bath)

Kraxen stove®

This is a modern adaptation of a tradition in the Alpine area
of Austria designed by the company Haslauer GmbH. The
name is derived from *kraxe*, a basket for the back that was
used to carry hay down the mountain by Alpine farmers. It
was also used in the living room of farmhouses where it was
placed near the stove to release the spice-scented aroma. In
the spa you sit with your back to the slatted wooden basket
filled with Alpine hay, free of pesticides and pollutants.
Steam is passed through the basket, releasing the pungent
characteristic odour of hay, resulting in a nurturing warm
feeling helping posture and relaxing the body.

Soft Pack system or Dry Float

Read the treatment card on page 81 'The Use and
Application of the Dry Float'.

The Use and Application of the Thermarium
Sauna and Saunarium
By: Jane Crebbin-Bailey HCB Associates

Benefit of treatment

A Finnish dry heat treatment in a wood-lined room. The heat induces sweating to cleanse the body of impurities. The sauna can operate as a saunarium with humidity automatically released into the air. The body gently heats up to stimulate the blood circulation which initiates the purifying and detoxifying process.

Advantages

- The temperature operates at 80°C – saunarium temperature operates at 60°C ambient air temperature with steam.
- Fully-tiled heated walls, floor and lounge benches seat 10 persons
- Fibre optic lighting
- Emergency call button

Contra-indications

- Skin diseases such as severe eczema or open psoriasis
- Cardiovascular disease (heart failure, coronary disease, strokes)
- Respiratory disease – severe asthma requiring regular inhaler use
- Pregnancy (not in the first four months)
- Client feels unwell with a fever
- High/low blood pressure
- Infected skin wounds
- Uncontrolled epilepsy

Preparation

- Operator/reception – First part of the day – Turn on system as per manufacturer's instructions (see 'Daily Operating Instructions Card')
- Fill the sauna bucket with a few drops of sauna essence and add fresh water. NEVER take the sauna essence into the sauna or allow guests to handle the bottle of essence, as the liquid is highly inflammable. NB undiluted essences are one of the major causes of fires in saunas
- Check the lights and fibre optic lights are operating
- Place the floor mats back in the correct position
- Place the bucket of water and diluted essence back in the sauna and ensure the ladle is to hand
- Add 2 ladles from the bucket on to the black filler located behind the top bench above the heaters. This will humidify the sauna

- Ensure client showers and hand them a towel and pair of slippers

Method

The sauna/saunarium should be included as part of a sequence:

- Show guests how to ladle the essence water in order to create steam in the sauna
- Guests should relax on their towel on the heated benches
- As the body heats, it will perspire. Rinse the body with the Kneipp hose (cool water) to refresh the body and stimulate the circulation
- Duration of 20 minutes
- Shower after the caldarium with cold or warm water
- Rest for 20 minutes before returning to the caldarium, laconium, hydro pool or other treatment involved in a sequence

After care

- Rest for about 20 minutes, preferably in a warm gown on a recliner
- Drink several glasses of still water
- Apply a good moisturiser to the skin after a shower or follow on with another treatment

Maintenance

- Read 'Daily Operating Instructions Card'. Ensure that the sauna is switched off at night
- Clean the floor and seating area with a suitable disinfectant
- Operate disinfecting cleansing system each night
- Check cleanliness of area on a regular basis – towels, floor, seating area, etc.
- Check fibre optic lighting is operating correctly
- Remove the floor mats and clean them
- Leave the sauna door open at night to allow it to dry out – this is important for the timber
- The sauna system will automatically shut down after 12 hours of heating

www.spa-therapy.com   ©HCB Associates – Mar 2001

The Use and Application of the Thermarium Tyrolean Sauna

By: Jane Crebbin-Bailey HCB Associates

Benefit of treatment

A Finnish dry heat treatment in a wood-lined room. The heat induces sweating to cleanse the body of impurities. The body gently heats up to stimulate the blood circulation, which initiates the purifying and detoxifying process.

Advantages

- The temperature operates at 80°C
- Emergency call button

Contra-indications and precautions

- Skin diseases such as severe eczema or open psoriasis
- Cardiovascular disease (heart failure, coronary disease, strokes)
- Respiratory disease – severe asthma requiring regular inhaler use
- Pregnancy (not in the first four months)
- Client feels unwell with a fever
- High/low blood pressure
- Infected skin wounds
- Uncontrolled epilepsy

Preparation

- Operator/reception – First part of the day – Turn on system as per manufacturer's instructions (see 'Daily Operating Instructions Card')
- Fill the sauna bucket with water
- Check the lights and fibre optic lights are operating
- Place the floor mats back in the correct position
- Place the bucket of water back in the sauna and ensure the ladle is to hand
- Add 5 ladles from the bucket on to the coals. This will humidify the sauna
- Ensure client showers and hand them a towel and pair of slippers

Method

The sauna/saunarium should be included as part of a sequence:

- Show guests how to ladle the essence water in order to create steam in the sauna
- Guests should relax on their towel on the heated benches
- Explain to clients that they MUST NOT place their towels near the sauna oven
- Duration of 20 minutes, shower or use the ice grotto after 10 minutes

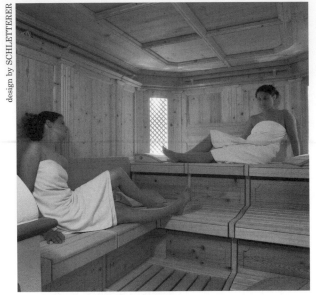

design by SCHLETTERER

www.berghof-zermatt.ch

- Shower after the sauna with cold water or cool mist experience shower
- Rest for 20 minutes before returning to spa experience involved in a sequence, or return to the sauna

After care

- Rest for about 20 minutes, preferably in a warm gown on a couch
- Drink several glasses of water
- Apply a good moisturiser to the skin after a shower or follow on with another treatment

Maintenance

- Read 'Daily Operating Instructions Card'. Ensure that the sauna is switched off at night
- Clean the floor and seating area with a suitable disinfectant
- Check cleanliness of area on a regular basis – towels, floor, seating area, etc.
- Constantly check that clients are not placing towels near the oven
- Remove the floor mats (optional accessory) and clean them
- Leave the sauna door open at night to allow it to dry out – this is important for the timber
- The sauna system will automatically shut down after 12 hours of heating

www.spa-therapy.com

©HCB Associates – Mar 2001

The Use and Application of the Thermarium Laconium

By: Jane Crebbin-Bailey HCB Associates

Benefit of treatment

A relaxing dry aromatic environment creating a Roman sauna atmosphere, with light and sound effects to stimulate the five senses. The purifying and detoxifying process is initiated by the body gently heating up to stimulate the blood circulation.

Advantages

- The temperature operates between 65°C, with 15–20% humidity, which is cooler than the traditional Finnish sauna
- Fully-tiled heated walls, floor and contoured lounge benches seats 6–8 persons
- Kniepp hose to refresh and cool the body enabling the client to spend longer periods in the laconium
- Automatic aromatic essence injector unit
- Fountain of water – to prevent static air build-up
- Emergency call button

Contra-indications and precautions

- Skin disease, such as severe eczema or open psoriasis
- Cardiovascular disease (heart failure, coronary disease, strokes)
- Respiratory disease – severe asthma requiring regular inhaler use
- Pregnancy (not in the first four months)
- Client feels unwell with a fever
- High/low blood pressure
- Infected skin wounds
- Uncontrolled epilepsy

Preparation

- Operator/reception – First part of the day – Turn on system as per manufacturer's instructions (see 'Daily Operating Instructions Card')
- Ensure client showers and hand them a towel and pair of slippers
- Explain to the client that the Kneipp hose can be used to rinse the seating area prior and after a treatment

Method

The laconium should be included as part of a sequence:

- Relax on the heated ceramic couches – place your feet on the tiled centre foot rest

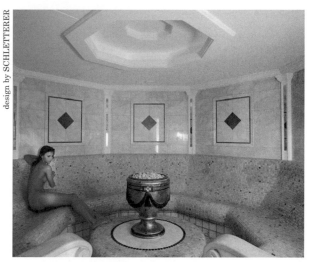

design by SCHLETTERER

www.vitalhotel-edelweiss.at

- As the body heats, it will perspire. Rinse the body with the Kneipp hose (cool water) to refresh the body and stimulate the circulation
- Duration of 20 minutes
- Shower after the laconium with cold or warm water
- Rest for 20 minutes before either returning to the laconium, Turkish hamman, hydro pool or other treatment involved in a sequence

After care

- Rest for about 20 minutes, preferably in a warm gown on a recliner
- Drink several glasses of still water
- Apply a good moisturiser to the skin after a shower

Maintenance

- Clean seating area and Laconium with a disinfectant suitable for ceramic tiles
- Read 'Daily Operating Instructions Card'
- Operate disinfecting cleansing system each night
- Check cleanliness of area on a regular basis – towels, floor, seating area, etc.
- Check level of 'essence' bottles

The Use and Application of the Thermarium
Caldarium – Mild Steam Room

By: Jane Crebbin-Bailey HCB Associates

Benefit of treatment

Based upon a Roman-style steam room with an aromatic moist atmosphere to either relax or stimulate the client, with light and sound effects to stimulate the five senses. The body gently heats up to stimulate the blood circulation which initiates the purifying and detoxifying process.

Advantages

- The temperature operates between 42–45°C – ambient air temperature with steam
- Fully-tiled heated walls, floor and lounge benches seats 10 persons
- Kniepp hose to refresh and cool the body enabling the client to spend longer periods in the caldarium
- Selection of electronically injected aromatic essences with steam – lavender, rose, jasmine and summer-meadow
- Fibre optic lighting or painted ceiling
- Emergency call button

Contra-indications and precautions

- Skin disease, such as severe eczema or open psoriasis
- Cardiovascular disease (heart failure, coronary disease, strokes)
- Respiratory disease – severe asthma requiring regular inhaler use
- Pregnancy (not in the first four months)
- Client feels unwell with a fever
- High/low blood pressure
- Infected skin wounds
- Uncontrolled epilepsy

Preparation

- Operator/reception – First part of the day – Turn on system as per manufacturer's instructions (see 'Daily Operating Instructions Card')
- Ensure client showers and hand them a towel and pair of slippers
- Explain to the client that the Kniepp hose can be used to rinse the seating area prior to and after a treatment

Method

The caldarium should be included as part of a sequence:

- Relax on a towel on the heated ceramic lounges

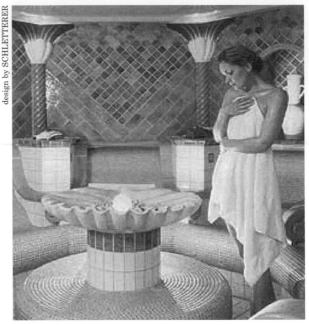

design by SCHLETTERER

www.thermarium.com

- As the body heats it will perspire. Rinse the body with the Kneipp hose (cool water) to refresh the body and stimulate the circulation
- Duration of 20 minutes
- Shower after the caldarium with cold or warm water
- Rest for 20 minutes before either returning to the caldarium, laconium, hydro pool or other treatment involved in a sequence

After care

- Rest for about 20 minutes, preferably in a warm gown on a recliner
- Drink several glasses of still water
- Apply a good moisturiser to the skin after a shower or follow on with another treatment

Maintenance

- Clean seating area and caldarium with a disinfectant suitable for ceramic tiles
- Read 'Daily Operating Instructions Card'
- Operate disinfecting cleansing system each night
- Check cleanliness of area on a regular basis – towels, floor, seating area, etc.
- Check level of essence bottles
- Check fibre optic lighting is operating correctly

The Use and Application of the Thermarium
Turkish Hamman

By: Jane Crebbin-Bailey HCB Associates

Benefit of treatment

Based upon a Roman-style steam room with an aromatic moist atmosphere to relax the client, with light and sound effects to stimulate the five senses. The body heats up to stimulate the blood circulation which initiates the purifying and detoxifying process.

Advantages

- The temperature operates between 60–80°C – ambient air temperature with steam
- Fully-tiled heated walls, floor and lounge benches, seats 10 persons
- Kniepp hose to refresh and cool the body enabling the client to spend longer periods in the Turkish hamman
- Electronically injected aromatic essences with steam – eucalyptus
- Fibre optic lighting
- Emergency call button

Contra-indications and precautions

- Skin disease, such as severe eczema or open psoriasis
- Cardiovascular disease (heart failure, coronary disease, strokes)
- Respiratory disease – severe asthma requiring regular inhaler use
- Pregnancy (not in the first four months)
- Client feels unwell with a fever
- High/low blood pressure
- Infected skin wounds
- Uncontrolled epilepsy

Preparation

- Operator/reception – First part of the day – Turn on system as per manufacturer's instructions (see 'Daily Operating Instructions Card')
- Ensure client showers and hand them a towel and pair of slippers
- Explain to the client that the Kneipp hose can be used to rinse the seating area prior and after a treatment

Method

The Turkish hamman should be included as part of a Sequence:

- As the body heats, it will perspire. Rinse your body with the Kneipp hose (cool water) to refresh the body and stimulate the circulation
- Duration of 20 minutes

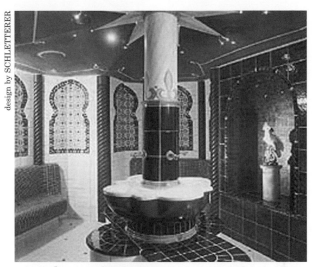

design by SCHLETTERER

www.thermarium.com

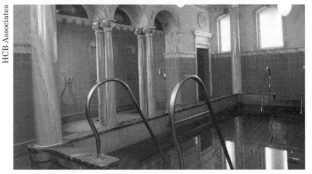

HCB Associates

Turkish Hamman, Sturabadet, Sweden

- Shower after the Turkish hamman with cold or warm water or use the ice room
- Rest for 20 minutes before either returning or moving on to another spa experience involved in a sequence

After care

- Rest for about 20 minutes, preferably in a warm gown on a recliner
- Drink several glasses of still water
- Apply a good moisturiser to the skin after a shower or follow on with another treatment

Maintenance

- Clean seating area and Turkish hamman with a disinfectant suitable for ceramic tiles
- Read 'Daily Operating Instructions Card'
- Check cleanliness of area on a regular basis – towels, floor, seating area, etc.

www.spa-therapy.com

The use and application of the Thalatherm
By: Jane Crebbin-Bailey HCB Associates

Benefit of treatment

An aromatic steam capsule with tropical rain shower. The client is enveloped with a suitable product chosen from cream/milk/seaweed or clay, whilst enjoying an aromatic gentle steam to provide the ultimate relaxation treatment, which is completed by a warm tropical rain shower and body moisturiser.

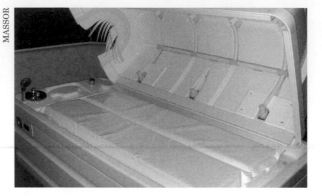

MASSOR

Advantages

- Multiple treatment use
- Shower network integrated in the dome, allowing complete body rinsing
- Hygienic and easy to clean
- Non-claustrophobic
- Can treat clients with mobility problems – easy access on to the table

Contra-indications

- Pregnancy (not in the first four months)
- Skin diseases, such as severe eczema or open psoriasis

Preparation

- During the first start-up, lift the dome lid and fill the steam outlets with water for 3 minutes. Then close the lid
- Adjust the steam generator thermostat – set the temperature according to client's needs and products used, generally between 34–38°C
- Set the timer to required treatment time, a green light will show
- Steam infusion starts about 30 seconds after start up. The thermostat detector records the temperature and automatically adjusts to the chosen setting
- Lift out the cartridge from the aromatherapy diffuser, sprinkle about 20 drops of a water soluble essential oil onto the absorbent part of the cartridge. Do not overload the cartridge. It is advisable to reserve one cartridge per aromatic used. Place the cover over the cartridge

Product use

Suitable creams/clays/seaweeds/milks/aromatics, lavender or hay pack

Please check with product manufacturer's guidelines for further contra-indications

Method

- Assist the client onto the thalatherm, ensure that the client's head is clear of the dome
- The client could have an exfoliation treatment at this stage prior to an envelopment or aromatic treatment. Use the hand held hose to rinse the client
- Apply your chosen treatment
- Pull down the dome lid and set the timer for 15 or 20 minutes. Adjust the head cushion to the client's comfort
- Keep checking on your client's comfort; wipe their face with a tissue if they perspire a lot
- When the machine has stopped, turn the tropical rain shower lever to position **A** for 20 seconds

This allows the existing water in the pipes to clear and the water to reach its thermostatic temperature
Never turn the lever to position **A** before the machine has stopped
- Turn the lever to position **B**. The Tropical rain shower now rinses the client. Allow 2 minutes. Its advisable to progressively decrease the temperature of the thermostat to about 30°C, in order to prevent too great a contrast of temperature when the dome is raised
- Turn the tropical rain shower lever to **C** (off)
- Slowly raise the lid of the dome, advising the client they will feel a slight draft of cool air, which is refreshing
- Help the client to sit up. Turn on the hand-held shower, firstly away from the client, to reach the desired temperature, then rinse the client's back
- The showerhead is fitted with 3 positions, adjustable with your thumb
  1. *Rain jet* (large diffusion of jets) advised at the end of rinsing
  2. *Concentrated jet.* Powerful, for cleaning off the Thalatherm
  3. *Foaming jet* (mixed with air). Perfect for rinsing the body
- Place a bathrobe or towel around your client and help them off the thalatherm
- The client is now ready for a follow-on treatment

After care

- Rest for about 20 minutes, preferably in a warm gown on a recliner
- Drink several glasses of still water
- Apply a good moisturiser to the skin after a shower

Maintenance

- The thalatherm has an acrylic coating. Use a specific cleaner for plastics, liquid soap with a slight detergent. NEVER use an abrasive pad or cleaning powder. Rinse thoroughly
- Clean and dry the chrome shower heads daily
- To disinfect the pipes, use a gentle anti-bactericide product, into the mouth's flow and leave it overnight
- If the flow is too slow, check and clean the trap. This can be located at the foot end of the machine and can easily be removed

The Use and Application of the Thermarium Aromatic Herb Bath

By: Jane Crebbin-Bailey HCB Associates

Benefit of treatment

A very mild sauna with low humidity and fresh herbal aromatic steam. Provides a gentle warm, scented mountain herb atmosphere. Relaxing and soporific, suitable for everyone as the preface to the complete spa experience.

Advantages

- The temperature operates at 60°C
- Fully-tiled heated walls, floor and seats in individual alcove
- Automatic disinfecting routine (optional)
- Emergency call button

Contra-indications and precautions

- Skin diseases, such as severe eczema or open psoriasis
- Cardiovascular disease (heart failure, coronary disease, strokes)
- Respiratory disease – severe asthma requiring regular inhaler use
- Pregnancy (not in the first four months)
- Client feels unwell with a fever
- High/low blood pressure
- Infected skin wounds
- Uncontrolled epilepsy

Preparation

- Operator/reception – First part of the day – Turn on the system as per manufacturer's instructions (see 'Daily Operating Instructions Card')
- Place fresh herbs on the tray every day – chamomile, rosemary, lavender or salvia (sage)
- Guest takes a shower

Method

- The central bucket of water turns on to the tray of warming herbs periodically, to create a mountain herb aromatic atmosphere
- This action takes 10 seconds and will slightly increase the temperature of the room. This action is repeated every 7 minutes per herb tray. In a session of 20 minutes the client will experience all three herbs
- Use the Kneipp hose (optional accessory) to cool the body down after about 10 minutes
- Guests leave the aromatic herbal bath after 20 – 30 minutes to rest in the relaxation area or continue on with another spa experience

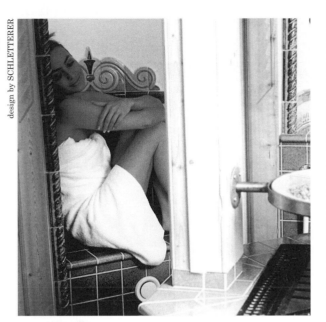

design by SCHLETTERER

www.adula.ch

After care

- Rest for about 20 minutes, preferably in a warm gown on a recliner
- Drink several glasses of still water
- Apply a good moisturiser to the skin after a shower

Maintenance

- Read 'Daily Operating Instructions Card'
- Clean the aromatic herbal bath with a disinfectant suitable for ceramic tiles
- Please ensure that the floor is kept clean and dry surrounding the aromatic herbal bath. Clean all corner areas of the floor with a high pressure hose and disinfectant each night
- Check cleanliness of area on a regular basis – towels, floor area, etc.
- Leave the door open at night to allow the room to ventilate

www.spa-therapy.com

This is a complete and virtually instant relaxation treatment where the body is cocooned in an occlusive waterproof sheet and suspended in warm water. The client floats in water, yet remains perfectly dry, except for any applications to the skin. This is a multi-use treatment ranging from a pre-heat treatment prior to a massage, to being enveloped in one of many different products that relax, detoxify, soothe, calm or energise the body and mind.

The following is a selection of typical treatments carried out with the Soft Pack system or Dry Float:

- mudpack
- peat
- fango pack
- Alpine hay
- wine therapy (you even get a glass of Chardonnay or Merlot to drink)
- algae (thalassotherapy)
- Rügen chalk (cleansing)
- salt (detoxifying and exfolient)
- evening primrose cream (for neuro-dermatitis and irritating skin disorders)
- Cleopatra (asses' milk, honey and essential oils).

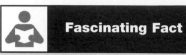
Fascinating Fact

Any special waterproof wrapping over the medicaments is called an occlusive dressing in medical circles. It has been recognised in medicine for sometime that these dressings open up the skin pores and facilitate the absorption of therapeutic substances.

Rasul

Read the treatment card on page 83, 'The Use and Application of the Rasul'.

The Rasul was developed from an ancient Arab cleansing and bathing ritual. Rasuls were installed in sultans' palaces for the harem. The Rasul combines the use of different muds to cleanse, absorb toxins and exfoliate the skin.

A medicinal earth from Greece – Terra Sealilata from the island of Limnos – was originally used. It is found in the veins of a mountain from this island and was also used for stamping a seal on a document, hence the name Terra Sealilata. This mud cannot be used today as the pH would be considered too acidic. Remember that people in the fifteenth century only used to bathe perhaps once a month, so their skin could tolerate these muds and there was a lot of dirt to remove!

Nowadays, muds are found all over the world with differing medicinal properties. Generally a cocktail of three muds is used in the Rasul. The muds are chosen for their different grain size and used on different parts of the

The Use and Application of the Dry Float Soft Pack System

By: Jane Crebbin-Bailey HCB Associates

Benefit of treatment

A complete and virtually instant relaxation treatment, where the body is cocooned in a waterproof sheet and literally dry floats, with no pressure points on the body, suspended in warm water.

Advantages

- Ergonomic – no pressure points on the body
- Multiple treatment use
- Can be used as a pre-heat treatment prior to massage for instance
- Hygienic

Contra-indications and precautions

- Claustrophobia
- Severe varicose veins
- Heart conditions (as heart failure, coronary disease, strokes)
- Skin diseases, such as severe eczema or open psoriasis
- Low blood pressure
- Uncontrolled epilepsy

Please check with product manufacturer's guidelines for further contra-indications

Preparation

- During the night the heating equipment is used as a preparation unit to warm the various mud, creams and liquids required for the following day's treatments
- The temperature of the bed is set to 34–38°C

Product use

- Muds and sea salts
- Fango mud and peat
- Herbs and hay
- Creams
- Liquids and milks
- Aromatics
- Seaweeds

Method

- Assist your client on to the bed
- Mud, algae and other pastes are spread directly over the body
- Liquids (milk) are soaked into two non-woven sheets. The client is between the sheets
- The client is wrapped in the waterproof sheet

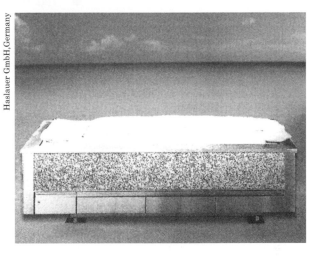

Haslauer GmbH, Germany

- The platform is lowered to create the sensation of floating
- The client should not be exposed to sudden temperature changes during the treatment
- The client relaxes for approximately 20 minutes depending upon the treatment, listening to music, or alternatively receives a scalp or face massage
- Raise the platform, fold back the waterproof sheet, place a bathrobe or towel around your client, help them off the bed and assist them to the shower

After care

- Rest for about 20 minutes, preferably in a warm gown on a recliner
- Drink several glasses of still water
- Apply a good moisturiser to the skin after a shower if appropriate

Maintenance

- Sanitise the waterproof sheet with a suitable product
- Stretch the waterproof sheet as it raises to minimise wrinkles in the fabric, and fold back neatly
- As the water is sealed in a waterproof folio, there is no need for filtration or purification systems

body – fine for the face to rough for the back – depending on their exfoliating properties. For example:

- *white bolus alpha* – for the face and sensitive parts of the body.
- *red bolus gamma* – for the front of body and arms.
- *blue/grey bolus epsilon* – for legs and back.

Salt is also used in this treatment for disinfecting the skin and, when applied to the back along the spinal column, is said to stimulate sweating. This treatment is contra-indicated in cases of psoriasis or eczema.

Clients sit in the Rasul, generally as couples or as a group, and the ceremony begins. Mud is applied to the body and the participants recline in ceramic seats – the entire body relaxes within seconds. Shots of steam blow through a bed of dried herbs and high quality essential oils, gradually increasing the humidity and temperature of the room. The highest temperature is 42°C. Unlike in a **steam room**, the body has time to adjust to the increasing temperature and humidity. As the mud bakes on the skin the client gently massages the skin. After 20 minutes an automatic shower of warm water is released from the planetarium ceiling rinsing off most of the mud from the body. The client leaves the Rasul and showers off the remainder of the mud in the antechamber and applies oil to nourish the skin. This treatment can be followed with a Cleopatra milk bath in the Dry Float bed.

Sand therapy (Psammo)

Sand baths are a type of thermal treatment using sea sand, including its salts and organic matter. It is also known as Psammo therapy where the approach is more medical. It is used for rheumatic and arthritic conditions and breathing difficulties. The client is wrapped in linen and placed in a bath of warm sand that moulds around the body. The temperature is the same as that of **fango** mud, but as the client is wrapped in linen (for hygienic reasons) there is no direct heat on the skin. The warmth of the sand induces relaxation, penetrates the muscles, benefiting the client.

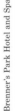

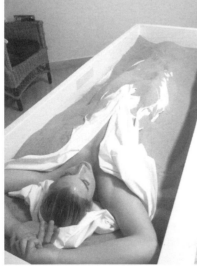

Psammo, Brenner's Park Hotel and Spa, Baden-Baden, Germany

Japanese enzyme bath (sometimes known as cedar bath)

This bath is used for relaxation and to reduce inflammation. It consists of a large redwood tub filled with cedar fibres and rice bran. These ingredients include over 600 enzymes and naturally ferment producing a cedar-

The Use and Application of the Rasul
By: Jane Crebbin-Bailey HCB Associates

Benefit of treatment

A relaxing therapeutic cleansing ceremony in a herbal gentle steam environment, combining different muds to cleanse, absorb toxins and exfoliate, increase circulation and leave the skin soft. Enhanced by light and sound effects to stimulate the five senses.

Advantages

- The temperature operates at an optimum working temperature 42°C
- Fully-tiled heated walls, floor
- Ergonomic seats for 2 persons or more
- Relaxing planetarium night sky ceiling
- Kneipp hose, located in each personal heated alcove to cool the body
- Automatic body and room showering system in ceiling
- Automatic aromatic steam injector unit that infuses a bed of dried herbs, increasing the ambient air temperature
- Emergency call button

Contra-indications and precautions

- Skin diseases, such as severe eczema or open psoriasis
- Cardiovascular disease (heart failure, coronary disease, strokes)
- Respiratory disease – severe asthma requiring regular inhaler use
- Pregnancy (not in the first four months)
- Client feels unwell with a fever
- High/low blood pressure
- Infected skin wounds
- Uncontrolled epilepsy

Preparation

- Operator/reception – First part of the day – Turn on the system as per manufacturer's instructions (see 'Daily Operating Instructions Card')
- Guest takes a shower
- In the antechamber, a trained spa attendant will advise guests on application of the mud to the body:
  - *white bolus alpha* – for the face and sensitive parts of the body
  - *red bolus gamma* – for the front of body and arms
  - *blue/grey bolus epsilon* – for legs and back

Method

- On entering the Rasul, the pre-heated air is dry to allow the guest to acclimatise to the aromatic herbal atmosphere
- The guest applies the various coloured muds to different areas of the body in a thin layer: steam and herbal essences are injected into the chamber and the temperature will rise to a maximum of 42°C. The duration is 20 minutes. The mud mask will start to dry on the skin. Check that the guest is comfortable
- Guests will massage the mud on their body with circular movements to facilitate the exfoliation of dead skin cells and elimination of toxins
- Guests will start to perspire in the herbal steam and can refresh themselves with the Kneipp hose
- After the programmed time of 20 minutes the herbal steam will start to clear and the automatic showering system will start. Advise the guests to remove as much of the mud as possible prior to leaving the room

- An optional shower may be taken in the spa
- Guests leaving the Rasul should be advised to rest in the relaxation area or tepidarium
- As an alternative treatment, the guest could experience a nourishing Cleopatra bath (milk, oil and honey) in the Soft Pack or Dry Float bed
- Once all the guests have left the room the spa attendant can activate the cleaning cycle (see maintenance)

After care

- Rest for about 20 minutes, preferably in a warm gown on a recliner
- Drink several glasses of still water
- Apply a good moisturiser to the skin after a shower

Maintenance

- After the client leaves the Rasul and ante-room, first remove any towels and mud bowls and close the door
- Switch on the cleaning light (red) with a key, in the panel. This activates the high pressure cleansing system which takes 4 minutes
- Dry the area and allow time for the temperature to increase prior to next client
- Clean seating area and Rasul with a disinfectant suitable for cleaning ceramic tiles

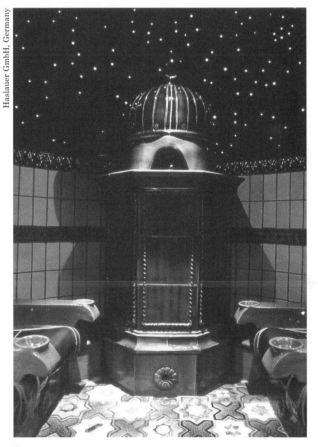

Haslauer GmbH, Germany

www.spa-therapy.com

©HCB Associates – June 2002

The Use and Application of the Thermarium Serail Mud Chamber

By: Jane Crebbin-Bailey HCB Associates

Benefit of treatment

A relaxing therapeutic cleansing ceremony in a herbal gentle steam environment, using therapeutic muds to exfoliate dead skin cells, eliminate toxins, increase circulation and leave the skin soft. Enhanced by light and sound effects to stimulate the five senses.

Advantages

- The temperature operates at between 35–45°C
- Fully-tiled heated walls, floor and alcove bench seats, for 2 persons or more
- Individual side body jets and Kneipp hose, located in each personal heated alcove
- Automatic aromatic essence injector unit – jasmine essence
- Emergency call button

Contra-indications and precautions

- Skin diseases, such as severe eczema or open psoriasis
- Cardiovascular disease (heart failure, coronary disease, strokes)
- Respiratory disease – severe asthma requiring regular inhaler use
- Pregnancy (not in the first four months)
- Client feels unwell with a fever
- High/low blood pressure
- Infected skin wounds
- Uncontrolled epilepsy
- Serious illness in the last 5 years

Preparation

- Operator/reception – First part of the day – Turn on the system as per manufacturer's instructions (see 'Daily Operating Instructions Card')
- Guest takes a shower
- In the antechamber, a trained spa attendant will advise guests on application of the mud to the body

Method

- On entering the Serail, the pre-heated air is dry
- After application of the mud, the spa attendant will check after 10 minutes that the mud is drying on the guest's skin. The spa attendant can then operate the steam by opening the panel with a key and pressing the 'steam on' button (**green**)
- Steam and herbal essences are injected into the chamber and the temperature will rise to a maximum of 45°C. The duration is 15 minutes. The mud mask will become supple. Check that the guest is comfortable
- Guests will massage the mud on their body with circular movements to facilitate the exfoliation of dead skin cells and elimination of toxins
- Guests will start to perspire in the herbal steam and can refresh themselves with the Kneipp hose, or approach

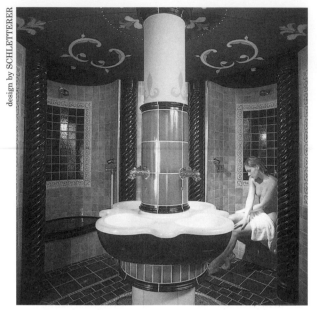

design by SCHLETTERER

www.trofana.at

the central basins to cool down by placing their hands under the central spout that will start automatically
- After the programmed time of 15 minutes the herbal steam will start to clear and guests will shower using the individual body jets – starting with the 'head shower' (30 seconds) followed by the 'side shower' (30 seconds). Advise the guests to remove as much of the mud as possible prior to leaving the room
- An optional shower may be taken in the spa
- Guests leaving the Serail mud chamber should be advised to rest in the relaxation area or tepidarium
- Once all the guests have left the room the spa attendant can activate the cleaning cycle (see maintenance)

After care

- Rest for about 20 minutes, preferably in a warm gown on a recliner
- Drink several glasses of still water
- Apply a good moisturiser to the skin after a shower

Maintenance

- After the client leaves the Serail and ante-room, first remove any towels and mud bowls and close the door
- Switch on the cleaning light (red) with a key, in the panel. This activates the high pressure cleansing system which takes 4 minutes
- Dry the area and allow time for the temperature to increase prior to next client
- Clean seating area and Serail mud chamber with a disinfectant suitable for cleaning ceramic tiles

www.spa-therapy.com

The Use and Application of the Thermarium
Japanese Salt Room

By: Jane Crebbin-Bailey HCB Associates

Benefit of treatment

A rose quartz crystal sits in the centre of the room with an automatic salt spray system. Humidity, essential oils and salt create an artificial sea atmosphere that opens the sinuses and clears the air passages. With heated seats and centre footrests. It is recommended that clients shower immediately after using the Japanese salt room before using any of the other spa experiences, to remove the salt from the skin, which could be drying.

Advantages

- The temperature operates between 45–48°C – ambient air temperature
- Fully-tiled heated walls, floor and lounge benches, seats 6 persons
- Individual seats with arm rests and central foot rest
- Electronically injected aromatic essences with steam (menthol, jasmine)
- Kneipp hose
- Emergency call button

Contra-indications and precautions

- Skin diseases, such as severe eczema or open psoriasis
- Cardiovascular disease (heart failure, coronary disease, strokes)
- Respiratory disease – severe asthma requiring regular inhaler use
- Pregnancy (not in the first four months)
- Client feels unwell with a fever
- High/low blood pressure
- Infected skin wounds
- Uncontrolled epilepsy

Preparation

- Operator/reception – First part of the day – Turn on system as per manufacturer's instructions (see 'Daily Operating Instructions Card')
- Ensure guest showers and hand them a towel and pair of slippers
- Optional but recommended: dry skin brushing with a loofah or natural bristle brush to prepare the skin for a steam treatment. This encourages the elimination of toxins and dead skin cells from the body

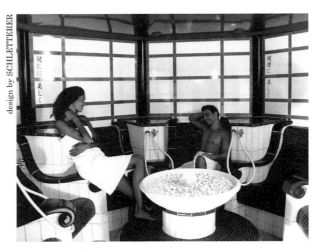

design by SCHLETTERER

www.schalber.com

Method

The Japanese salt room should be included as part of a sequence:

- Relax on the towel on the heated ceramic loungers
- Guest deeply inhales the salty air blended with the aroma of essential oils
- Duration of 15–20 minutes
- Shower after the Japanese salt room with cool or warm water
- Rest for 20 minutes before either returning to the tepidarium, caldarium, laconium, hydro pool or other treatment involved in a sequence

After care

- Rest for about 20 minutes, preferably in a warm gown on a recliner
- Drink several glasses of still water
- Apply a good moisturiser to the skin after a shower or follow on with another treatment

Maintenance

- Clean seating area Japanese salt room with a disinfectant suitable for ceramic tiles
- Read 'Daily Operating Instructions Card'
- Disinfect the ceramic seats
- Check cleanliness of area on a regular basis – towels, floor, seating area, etc.
- Check level of essence bottles
- Leave the door open at night to allow it to ventilate

www.spa-therapy.com

The Use and Application of the Thermarium Blossom Steam Room

By: Jane Crebbin-Bailey HCB Associates

Benefit of treatment

An Indian-style steam room with an aromatic moist atmosphere to relax or stimulate the client, with light and sound effects to stimulate the five senses. The body gently heats up to stimulate the blood circulation which initiates the purifying and detoxifying process.

Advantages

- The temperature operates between 42–45°C – ambient air temperature with steam
- Fully-tiled heated walls, floor and lounge, seats up to 10 persons
- Kniepp hose to refresh and cool the body enabling the client to spend longer periods in the Indian blossom steam room
- Selection of electronically-injected exotic aromatic essences with steam: ylang ylang
- Fibre optic lighting or painted ceiling
- Emergency call button

Contra-indications and precautions

- Skin diseases, such as severe eczema or open psoriasis
- Cardiovascular disease (heart failure, coronary disease, strokes)
- Respiratory disease – severe asthma requiring regular inhaler use
- Pregnancy (not in the first four months)
- Client feels unwell with a fever
- High/low blood pressure
- Infected skin wounds
- Uncontrolled epilepsy

Preparation

- Operator/reception – First part of the day – Turn on system as per manufacturer's instructions (see 'Daily Operating Instructions Card')
- Ensure client showers and hand them a towel and pair of slippers
- Explain to the client that the Kneipp hose can be used to rinse the seating area prior to and after a treatment

Method

The Indian blossom steam room should be included as part of a sequence:

- Relax on your towel on the heated ceramic loungers

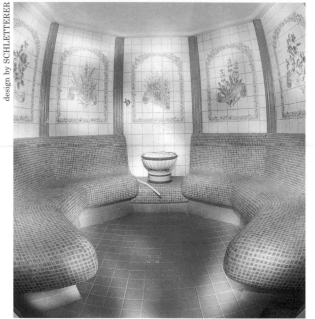

design by SCHLETTERER

www.thermarium.com

- As the body heats, it will perspire. Rinse the body with the Kneipp hose (cool water) to refresh the body and stimulate the circulation
- Duration of 20 minutes
- Shower after the Indian blossom steam room with cold or warm water
- Rest for 20 minutes before either returning to the caldarium, laconium, hydro pool or other treatment involved in a sequence

After care

- Rest for about 20 minutes, preferably in a warm gown on a recliner
- Drink several glasses of still water
- Apply a good moisturiser to the skin after a shower or follow on with another treatment

Maintenance

- Clean seating area and Indian blossom steam Room with a disinfectant suitable for ceramic tiles
- Read 'Daily Operating Instructions Card'
- Operate disinfecting cleansing system each night
- Check cleanliness of area on a regular basis – towels, floor, seating area, etc.
- Check level of essence bottles
- Check fibre optic lighting is operating correctly

scented hot steam that induces deep relaxation. Cool compresses are placed on the forehead. This bath is usually set in a garden of bonsai, bamboo and rock. After the bath the guest rests, wrapped in a robe or cotton blanket and either listens to music combined with natural sounds to relax brain-wave activity or strolls in the meditative Japanese garden. A green tea is often served to complete the treatment.

Zen garden

With time the artificial disappears and only the natural remains.

(Zen Buddhism saying)

Gardens of meditation and relaxation are becoming an integral and important part of today's spa. They provide an area for contemplation, for sitting silently watching everything come and go and allowing the mind to be free from unnecessary clutter. They offer a tranquil moment in harmony with nature, free from the busy urban life, to watch leaves fall and flowers bloom, listening to the bird song, touching and smelling the aromatic plants – treating the five senses.

Traditionally Zen gardens are minimalist, simple and spiritual with a courtyard, plain stone walls, raked gravel; they are kept free of weeds, with groups of rocks, water, stepping stones, a bamboo deer scarer and usually a wooden platform or veranda on which to sit and contemplate the garden. Zen gardens observe the natural landscape and allow nature to go where it wants to, combining natural (wood, stone) and man-made elements (glass, metal), subtle earth colours with perhaps the exception of one bloom that becomes a focus in the garden. This contrasts with Western gardens, which tend to be styled on symmetry, colour and flower beds.

Water has a symbolic meaning in the Zen garden where it is viewed as a journey through life and used in purification rituals. In a dry garden, an illusion of the flow of water can be created with light and dark gravel or carefully placed gravel and pebbles to represent the waves of the sea.

The harmony and balance in the Zen garden should allow the energy (*ki*) to flow freely. The symbols of balance are shown as yin and yang; the element yin is represented as sand and gravel, low shapes and shady areas and yang as rock and stone, tall, vertical shapes and sunny areas. The calm silence of the garden is yin and the sounds of nature, the wind through the branches and leaves, is yang. Yin and yang represent the two opposing forces of nature.

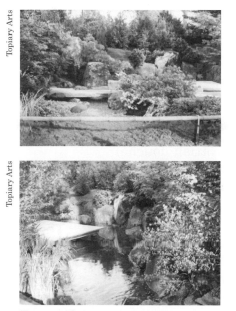

Zen gardens

Cold therapy treatments

Cold treatments are used for:

1. reducing the heat in hot inflamed joints

2. reducing swelling in joints and injured tissue

3. relieving pain in conditions 1 and 2 and through the analgesic effect on skin nerve endings.

Although peat can be used, loam is better because of its different thermophysical properties. With loam, heat loss is also increased due to evaporation. Loam quickly withdraws warmth from inflamed areas.

The Austrian company Haslauer GmbH produces a special cold pack for temperatures down to −20°C. This must be used with a protective sheet and for no longer than 4 minutes to avoid frostbite. The pack can be re-applied after 8 minutes.

Cryotherapy

This is also known as cryosurgery. It is a technique used by the medical profession to freeze and destroy a variety of benign skin growths, such as warts, pre-cancerous lesions – actinic keratoses and malignant lesions – basal cell and squamous cell cancers, and to preserve the surrounding skin tissue. The technique uses liquid nitrogen. The word 'cryotherapy' is sometimes misused in spa/beauty therapy by referring to cold applications.

Water therapy treatments

In this section, we will look at the following water therapy treatments:

● Japanese bathing
● Jet Blitz (douche a Jet/Scottish douche)
  Read treatment card on pages 92 and 93
  'The Use and Application of Jet/Scottish douche'
● Experience shower
  Read treatment Card on page 94, 'The Use and Application of the Experience Shower'
● Affusion shower
  Read treatment Card on pages 95 and 96, 'The Use and Application of Affusion/Vichy Shower'

The Use and Application of the Thermarium Ice Fountain

By: Jane Crebbin-Bailey HCB Associates

Benefit of treatment

A contrast to a heat treatment such as laconium or sauna. Stimulates the circulation, lymphatic and immune system. Is used in medical spas to treat anxiety, stress and depression.

Advantages

- Automatic release of ice through sensors
- The temperature operates at 15°C or less

Contra-indications and precautions

- Cardiovascular disease (heart failure, coronary disease, strokes)
- Respiratory disease – severe asthma requiring regular inhaler use
- Pregnancy (not in the first four months)
- Client feels unwell with a fever
- High/low blood pressure
- Infected skin wounds
- Uncontrolled epilepsy

Preparation

- Operator/reception – First part of the day – Turn on the system as per manufacturer's instructions (see 'Daily Operating Instructions Card')

Method

- Guests rub the crushed ice all over the body to cool it down, leaving a fresh and invigorating feeling
- Guests leave the Ice Fountain to rest in the relaxation area or continue on with another spa experience
- Rest for 20 minutes before either returning to the sauna, tepidarium, caldarium, laconium, hydro pool or other Spa experience involved in a sequence

After care

- Rest for about 20 minutes, preferably in a warm gown on a recliner
- Drink several glasses of water
- Apply a good moisturiser to the skin after a shower

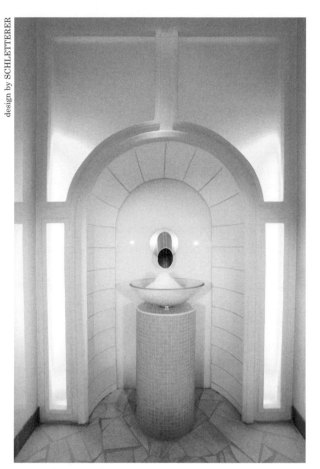

design by SCHLETTERER

www.thermarium.com

Maintenance

- Read 'Daily Operating Instructions Card'
- Clean the ice fountain with a disinfectant suitable for ceramic tiles
- Please ensure that the floor is kept clean and dry surrounding the ice fountain
- Check the sensors in the basin are not blocked with ice
- Check cleanliness of area on a regular basis – towels, floor area, etc.

The Use and Application of the Thermarium
Ice Room
By: Jane Crebbin-Bailey HCB Associates

Benefit of treatment

A contrast to a heat treatment such as laconium or sauna. Stimulates the circulation, lymphatic and immune system. Is used in medical spas to treat anxiety, stress and depression.

Advantages

- The temperature operates at 15°C or less
- Fully-tiled walls, floor and supporting bar to lean on
- Fibre optic lighting
- Air-conditioned room
- Emergency call button

Contra-indications and precautions

- Cardiovascular disease (heart failure, coronary disease, strokes)
- Respiratory disease – severe asthma requiring regular inhaler use
- Pregnancy (not in the first four months)
- Client feels unwell with a fever
- High/low blood pressure
- Infected skin wounds
- Uncontrolled epilepsy

Preparation

- Operator/reception – First part of the day – Turn on the system as per manufacturer's instructions (see 'Daily Operating Instructions Card')

Method

- Guests rub the crushed ice all over the body to cool it down, leaving a fresh and invigorating feeling
- Guests leave the Ice Grotto to rest in the relaxation area or continue on with another spa experience
- Rest for 20 minutes before either returning to the sauna, tepidarium, caldarium, laconium, hydro pool or other treatment involved in a sequence

After care

- Rest for about 20 minutes, preferably in a warm gown on a recliner
- Drink several glasses of water
- Apply a good moisturiser to the skin after a shower

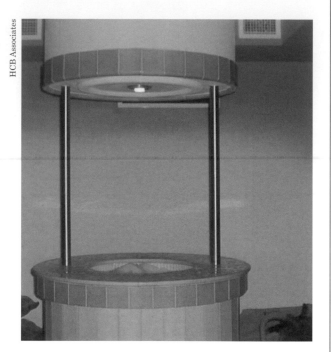
HCB Associates

Maintenance

- Read 'Daily Operating Instructions Card'
- Clean the ice grotto with a disinfectant suitable for ceramic tiles
- Please ensure that the floor is kept clean and dry surrounding the ice grotto
- Check cleanliness of area on a regular basis – towels, floor area, etc.
- Check fibre optic lighting is operating correctly
- Leave the door open at night to allow the room to ventilate

- Aqua meditation
  Read treatment card on page 97, 'The Use and Application of the Aqua Meditation'
- Chakra therapy room
  Read treatment card on page 98, 'The Use and Application of the Chakra Therapy Room'
- Pedidarium (reflexology basins)
  Read treatment card on page 99, 'The Use and Application of the Reflexology Basins'
- Cleopatra slipper bath
  Read treatment card on page 100, 'The Use and Application of the Cleopatra Slipper Bath'
- Hydro pool and hydrotherapy
  Read treatment card on page 101, 'The Use and Application of Hydro pools'
  Read treatment card on pages 102 and 103, 'The Use and Application of Hydrotherapy Baths'

Japanese bathing

The *ofuro* consists of a room with a central drain, a tub (bath), showering area, a sitting stool and wooden bucket. The tradition is to sit on the stool and wash the body with soap and sponges in circular movements towards the heart in a contemplative mood. The bucket is filled with warm water and poured over the body. These actions are repeated several times before showering and then soaking in the tub (bath). The public bathhouse, *osento*, was traditionally built near **hot mineral springs**, nowadays many of them are a part of a theme park.

Massage

Different massage therapies have evolved around the world over many centuries, for stress, muscle and tissue relaxation as well as manipulation of the skin, muscles and joints.

Deep (tissue) muscle massage

A deep muscle massage helps to realign the body and give freedom of movement. This can be an uncomfortable massage for the client as it separates muscle groups and connective tissue to improve posture and give relief of chronic tensions.

The Use and Application of the Jet/Scottish douche
By: Jane Crebbin-Bailey, HCB Associates

Benefit of treatment

The jet/Scottish douche, or Blitz as it is sometimes known, revitalises and energises the body by working on the circulatory systems. Standing at the end of a room, the therapist works the muscles with warm pressurised water, relieving tension and stress. These drainage techniques when performed with care, have excellent results on the lymphatic and circulatory systems.

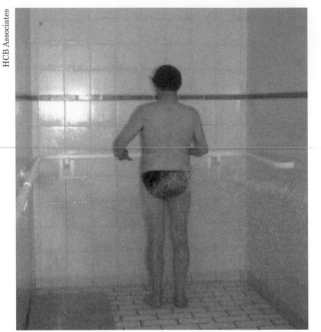

Advantages

- Good combination treatment e.g. with a massage/Rasul aromatic steam treatment – massortherm/Dry Float/affusion shower
- Energising
- 20-minute treatment

Contra-indications

- Pregnancy (not in the first three months)
- Heart conditions (heart failure, coronary disease, strokes)
- Skin diseases, such as severe eczema or open psoriasis
- Severe varicose veins (avoid jets on the lower limb)
- Respiratory disease – severe asthma requiring regular inhaler use
- Uncontrolled epilepsy
- Cancer
- Coil/menstruation (avoid the stomach area)
- Bruising
- Avoid the spine and areas of bone (i.e. hip joint area)
- Avoid crossing from the sigmoid colon to the ascending colon (stomach area)

Preparation

- Ensure that prior to the client entering the room the floor is dry
- Ensure that the water temperature is set to 34°C

Product use

- Hot and cold water supply or seawater

Method

Scottish douche – water techniques

- Care must be taken with the pressure and the direction of the hose
- Directional hose – using the pressure jet

- Tapping using a broken spray – alternating pressure jet and spray

Each action is performed in a series of three

- Assist your client to the end of the room
- Explain the procedure of the treatment to the client
- Complete the treatment by asking your client to continuously turn slowly around whilst you spray their whole body with tepid water

Please see: treatment card 'Lymphatic Drainage Techniques using the Jet/Scottish douche' opposite for a step-by-step guide to lymphatic drainage massage

After care

- Rest for about 20 minutes, preferably in a warm gown on a recliner
- Drink several glasses of water
- Apply a good moisturiser to the skin after a shower

Maintenance

- Dismantle and thoroughly clean shower heads every day

www.spa-therapy.com

Lymphatic Drainage Techniques
Using the Jet/Scottish douche
By: Jane Crebbin-Bailey, HCB Associates

Benefit of treatment

The jet/Scottish douche, or blitz as it is sometimes known, revitalises and energises the body by working on the circulatory systems. Standing at the end of a room, the therapist works the muscles with warm pressurised water, relieving tension and stress. These drainage techniques when performed with care, have excellent results on the lymphatic and circulatory systems.

Advantages

- Energising
- 20-minute treatment

Contra-indications

- Pregnancy (not in the first three months)
- Heart conditions (as heart failure, coronary disease, strokes)
- Skin diseases, such as severe eczema or open psoriasis
- Severe varicose veins (avoid jets on the lower limb)
- Respiratory disease – severe asthma requiring regular inhaler use
- Uncontrolled epilepsy
- Cancer
- Coil/menstruation (avoid the stomach area)
- Bruising
- Avoid the spine and areas of bone (i.e. hip joint area)
- Avoid crossing from the sigmoid colon to the ascending colon (stomach area)

Preparation

- Ensure that prior to the client entering the room the floor is dry
- Ensure that the water temperature is set to 34°C

Product use

- Hot and cold water supply or seawater

Method

Scottish douche – water techniques

- Care must be taken with the pressure and the direction of the hose
- Directional hose – using the pressure jet
- Tapping using a broken spray – alternating pressure jet and spray

Each action is performed in a series of three

- Assist your client to the end of the room
- The client stands facing the wall, holding the bars, with their legs slightly apart
- Explain the procedure of the treatment to the client

Back of body – right side

- Sole of foot – spiral clockwise up towards the heal
- Right leg – outer side of leg – start at the ankle and sweep up towards the hip and off towards the wall
- Inside leg – start at the ankle and up towards the knee, cross just under the buttock and continue up on outer side of thigh to hip
- Right buttock – spiral clockwise, keeping the spiral to a rugger ball shape

Back of body – left side

- Left foot – repeat anti-clockwise
- Left leg – repeat anti-clockwise

- Left buttock – repeat anti-clockwise

Back

- Right – start above the buttock up towards the shoulder blade, spiral clockwise on the shoulder blade
- Left – repeat anti-clockwise
- Bottom – triangle – clockwise between hips, starting from coccyx
- Top of back – triangle – clockwise between the shoulders
- The whole back – using the spray, form a figure of 8 from lower to upper back, sweep up and down

Body in profile – right profile

- Foot – turned towards you, tapping movement on top of the foot
- Ankle – circle clockwise around ankle bone
- Leg – from ankle to buttock
- Hip – clockwise on hip area
- Side of ribs – client's right arm protects breast area. Spray jet from hips to armpit, gentle sweep over same area. Lower arm back alongside body
- Hand – tapping jet on palm
         – tapping jet on top of hand
- Arm – clockwise from wrist to elbow, circle clockwise around the elbow, continue up from elbow to shoulder. Circle clockwise around shoulder

Body in profile – left profile

Repeat all of the above movements in an anti-clockwise direction

Client facing you – right side

- Foot – tapping jet on top of foot
- Leg – outer side of leg – sweep from ankle to hip
       – inside of leg – sweep from ankle to knee, continue to just above mid thigh, then cross to outer leg and finish at hip
- Hip – spiral clockwise, keeping the spiral to a rugger ball shape

Client facing you – left side

Repeat all of the above movements in an anti-clockwise direction

- Stomach – gentle pressure starting from the ascending colon across the transverse and down the descending to the sigmoid colon then gently sweep back in opposite direction with a spray movement. DO NOT cross from the sigmoid colon to the ascending colon
- Shoulder – ask your client to turn their head away from the direction of the hose
- Right – circle in a clockwise direction around the shoulder
- Left – circle in an anti-clockwise direction around the shoulder

To finish

Complete the treatment by asking your client to continuously turn slowly around whilst you spray their whole body with tepid water

After care

- Rest for about 20 minutes, preferably in a warm gown on a recliner
- Drink several glasses of water
- Apply a good moisturiser to the skin after a shower

Maintenance

- Dismantle and thoroughly clean shower heads every day

The Use and Application of the Experience Shower
By: Jane Crebbin-Bailey HCB Associates

Benefit of treatment

The experience shower has several options, from a cold fog mist combined with a mint essence to enhance a feeling of coolness after a heat treatment, to a cold mint rain. Alternatively, a tropical rain-like massage shower using passion fruit essence invigorates you prior to a heat treatment.

Advantages

- Side body jets and an overhead shower, to give an invigorating shower
- Automatically time controlled per shower experience
- Water saving – guest can only take one experience shower sequence at a time – duration approximately 2 minutes
- Hygienic and easy to clean
- Automatic aromatic essence injector unit and fibre optic lighting to stimulate the five senses
- Aromatic essence injector unit can alter volume and percentage

Contra-indications and precautions

- Skin diseases, such as severe eczema or open psoriasis
- Cardiovascular disease (heart failure, coronary disease, strokes)
- Respiratory disease – severe asthma requiring regular inhaler use
- Pregnancy (not in the first four months)
- Client feels unwell with a fever
- High/low blood pressure
- Infected skin wounds
- Uncontrolled epilepsy

Preparation

- Operator/reception – First part of the day – Turn on system as per manufacturer's instructions (see 'Daily Operating Instructions Card')
- Ensure client has a towel and pair of slippers

Method

The experience shower should be included as part of a sequence:

- The guest commences with a spa experience for 20 minutes then uses the shower in between the sequence
- Explain the use of the shower – A combination of 3 buttons *per* experience shower (2 cannot be pressed at the same time)

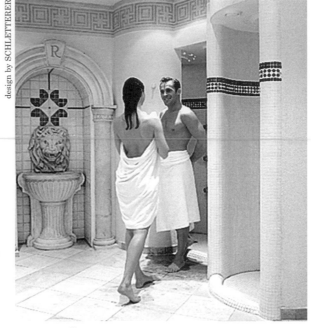

design by SCHLETTERER

www.trofana.at

1. Rain – Cold + mint
2. Tropical – Warm + passion fruit
3. Fresh – Cold mist + mint
4. Side – Warm, can be with a thermostatic mixer, no essence
5. Splash – Cold with 4–6 jets that create a film of water over the body – no essence
6. Head – shower head (not removable)

NB *Please note that this experience shower can be used as a treatment on its own*

After care

- Rest for about 20 minutes, preferably in a warm gown on a couch
- Drink several glasses of still water
- Apply a good moisturiser to the skin after a shower

Maintenance

- Read 'Daily Operating Instructions Card'
- Clean the experience shower with a disinfectant suitable for ceramic tiles
- Please ensure that the floor is kept clean and dry prior to the guest entering the room
- Check cleanliness of area on a regular basis – towels, floor area, etc.
- Check level of essence bottles

www.spa-therapy.com   ©HCB Associates – Mar 2001

The use and application of Affusion/Vichy Showers
By Jane Crebbin-Bailey HCB Associates

Benefit of treatment

Sedating, anti-stress massage under a warm tropical rain shower. The massage improves blood and lymph circulation, nourishes the skin and relaxes the nerves.

Advantages

- Very relaxing treatment
- Can treat clients with mobility problems – easy access on to the table
- Introduction to aromatics
- Gentle massage pressure on the body – can work on clients with varicose problems
- Dual system – manual lymphatic massage treatment or automatic aromatic shower

Contra-indications

- Pregnancy (not in the first three months)
- Skin diseases, such as severe eczema or open psoriasis

Preparation

- Ensure that prior to the client entering the room the floor is dry
- Ensure that the water temperature is set to 38°C
- Add the chosen aromatic to the diffuser

Product use

Aromatics – preferably water based for the filtration system

Method one

- Assist your client on to the massage table
- The client lies *face* down on a massage table suitable for wet treatments
- Move the face guard in front of the face
- Start the multiple shower away from the client and bring the shower arm across the client's body. Leave the client to relax for 10 minutes, where upon the body is massaged with warm droplets of aromatic rain
- After 10 minutes, move the shower arm and face guard away from the client's body and ask the client to turn over on to their back and bring the shower arm and face guard across the body for a further 10 minutes
- When the treatment has finished, turn off the shower, move the apparatus away from the client
- Place a bathrobe or towel around your client and help them off the massage table and assist the client to the relaxation room

Method two – using lymphatic massage techniques

- Assist your client on to the massage table
- The client lies *face* down on a massage table suitable for wet treatments
- Start the multiple shower and leave the client to relax for 5 minutes, whereupon the body is massaged with warm droplets of aromatic rain

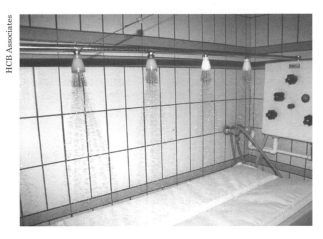

HCB Associates

- The massage is performed with passive movements:
  - The joints are massaged with *effleurage or stroking movements* with no resistance or assistance by muscular activity on the part of the client
  - The movements are divided into *superficial, feathering and deep*, over large surfaces, varying the amount of pressure. Generally the movement is towards the heart
- At the end of the massage, start the multiple shower and leave the client to relax for 5 minutes, whereupon the body is massaged with warm droplets of aromatic rain
- When the treatment has finished, turn off the shower, move the apparatus away from the client
- Place a bathrobe or towel around your client and help them off the massage table and assist the client to the relaxation room

Please see: step-by-step treatment card 'Lymphatic Drainage Techniques for Affusion Showers' overleaf for a visual guide to the massage

After care

- Rest for about 20 minutes, preferably in a warm gown on a recliner
- Drink several glasses of water
- Apply a good moisturiser to the skin

Maintenance

- Dismantle shower heads once a week and thoroughly clean
- Clean the aromatic filters
- Use a specific cleaner for plastics, liquid soap with a slight detergent. NEVER use an abrasive pad or cleaning powder
- Sanitise the waterproof sheet of the massage table with a suitable product

Lymphatic Drainage Techniques using Affusion Showers
By: Jane Crebbin-Bailey HCB Associates

Benefit of treatment

Anti-stress. Improves blood and lymph circulation, nourishes the skin and relaxes the nerves.
Your client lies on a massage table suitable for wet treatments under a multiple shower hose. He/she is then massaged with warm droplets of aromatic rain.

Method

- Your client lies face down on a massage table suitable for wet treatments
- Start the multiple shower and leave him/her to relax for 5 minutes, whereupon the body is massaged with warm droplets of aromatic rain
- The massage is performed with passive movements:
  - The joints are massaged with *effleurage or stroking movements* with no resistance or assistance by muscular activity on the part of your client
  - The movements are divided into *superficial, feathering and deep*, over large surfaces, varying the amount of pressure. Generally the movement is towards the heart

Foot. Start the massage by kneading the sole of the foot from the toes towards the heel, in circular movements. 3 times left then right foot

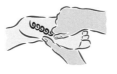

Leg. Stroke the leg upwards with both hands. 5 times. If there are particularly tight areas use more pressure with the heel of the hand.
Left then right leg

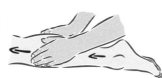

Thigh. Stroke the thigh up towards the buttocks. 5 times. Increasing the pressure with each upward stroke. Left then right thigh

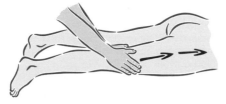

Back 1. Effleurage the back, starting at the base of the spine, with the little finger leading and the rest of the fingers pointing towards the spine. Move your hands out over the shoulders and return along the sides to the hips. 5 times, increasing the pressure with each upward stroke

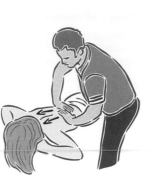

Back 2. Outward stretching of the muscles. 5 times

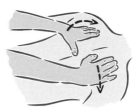

Back 3. Inward stretching of the muscles. 5 times

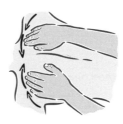

Back 4. Standing at your client's head, effleurage from the nape of the neck down towards the lower back, and return with slightly stronger pressure. 5 times

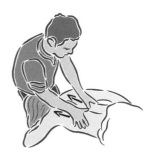

Back 5. Standing at the side of your client, stroke the back using fanning action downwards. 5 times

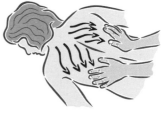

The Use and Application of the Thermarium Aqua Meditation Room

By: Jane Crebbin-Bailey HCB Associates

Benefit of treatment

The aqua meditation room has a large raised fountain in the centre of this tranquil relaxation room, and when droplets of water are released from the ceiling and hit the mirrored, lit fountain they send a ripple through the water that reflects up on to the ceiling. A relaxing, warm, dry aromatic environment with light and sound effects to stimulate the five senses. The guest relaxes on a cushioned relining bench looking up at the light reflected ripples of water on the ceiling whilst listening to calming music. Relax, reflect and contemplate. You can stay in this room for long periods and it is ideal prior to massage treatments or also (or between) the other heat experiences.

Advantages

- The temperature operates at 28°C – ambient air temperature
- Gently heated floor and ergonomic heated cushioned benches, seats up to 10 persons
- Lemon aromatic scent injector
- Automatic filling and emptying of water in base of fountain
- Emergency call button

Contra-indications and precautions

- Cardiovascular disease (heart failure, coronary disease, strokes)
- Respiratory disease – severe asthma requiring regular inhaler use
- Client feels unwell with a fever
- Infected skin wounds
- Uncontrolled epilepsy

Preparation

- Operator/reception – First part of the day – Turn on system as per manufacturer's instructions (see 'Daily Operating Instructions Card')
- Check the sound level of music

Method

The aqua meditation room should be included as part of a sequence:

- Relax in your towelling bath robe on the heated benches
- Rest for 20–30 minutes before returning to the caldarium, laconium, hydro pool or other treatment involved in a sequence

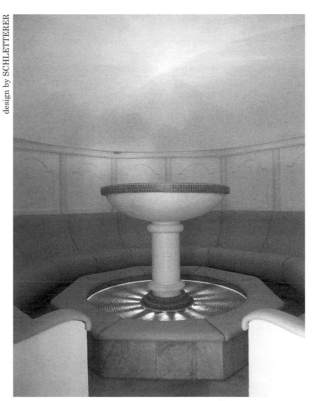

design by SCHLETTERER

www.thermarium.com

- Shower after the aqua meditation room with cold or warm water

After care

- Rest for about 20 minutes, preferably, in a warm gown on a recliner
- Drink several glasses of water
- Apply a good moisturiser to the skin after a shower or follow on with another treatment

Maintenance

- Read 'Daily Operating Instructions Card'
- Clean seating area of the leather-style heated benches with a suitable *proprietary* cleaner
- Check cleanliness of area on a regular basis – towels, floor, seating area, etc.
- Check level of 'essence' bottles
- Check water inlets in ceiling are operating correctly
- Clean mirrored glass in fountain
- Check light in fountain is operating

www.spa-therapy.com

©HCB Associates – July 2002

The Use and Application of the Chakra Therapy Room

By: Jane Crebbin-Bailey HCB Associates

Benefit of treatment

The skin is given a quick soft brush followed by a warm soap foam scrub to exfoliate the skin and remove toxins. The guest is dried and given a herbal drink before experiencing a warm oil massage incorporating the chakra points of the head and body performed by two therapists in an aromatic filled room with relaxing music to treat the five senses and totally relax the body.

Advantages

- Multiple treatment use – luxury treatment room with a multi-purpose use, often incorporating a hydro bath, slipper bath or steam room
- Shower network integrated in the table, allowing complete body rinsing
- Hygienic and easy to clean
- Can treat clients with mobility problems – easy access on to the table

Contra-indications

- Skin diseases, such as severe eczema or open psoriasis
- Cardiovascular disease (heart failure, coronary disease, strokes)
- Respiratory disease – severe asthma requiring regular inhaler use
- Pregnancy (not in the first four months)
- Client feels unwell with a fever
- High/low blood pressure
- Infected skin wounds
- Uncontrolled epilepsy

Preparation

- Operator/reception – First part of the day – Turn on system as per manufacturer's instructions (see 'Daily Operating Instructions Card')
- Pre-heat the chakra therapy table – automatically pre-set temperature of 37–38°C
- The room should be filled with Ayurvedic aromatic essences and therapeutic music
- The therapist assesses the guest in order to prepare the oil for the massage
- The oil temperature is 37–38°C

Method

The chakra therapy room should be included as part of a Sequence:

- The guest commences with a caldarium treatment for 10 minutes

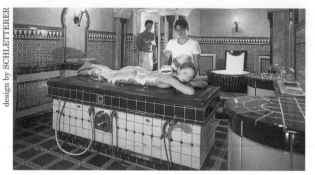

design by SCHLETTERER

www.trofana.at

- Shower and towel dries
- Assist the guest on to the chakra therapy table and give a quick soft dry massage
- Follow with a warm soap foam scrub, the soap/foam scrub shower unit is located on the side of the table
- Using the hand held shower, the guest is rinsed whilst still on the table
- Towel dry the guest
- Give the guest a herbal drink and rest for 20 minutes before performing the chakra massage
- A warm oil massage is given for 20–30 minutes concentrating on the chakra points. One or two therapists can administer the massage with one concentrating on a scalp and face massage, the other on the body
- The guest now rests with the anointed oil and is covered with foil and a blanket for 10 minutes
- Remove the foil and blanket
- The guest takes a final shower before relaxing on the heated ceramic relaxation couches for 20 minutes

NB *Please note that this therapy room may be used for other treatments – salt scrub, loofah soap scrub and other wet massage treatments*

After care

- Rest for about 20 minutes, preferably in a warm gown on a recliner
- Drink several glasses of still water
- Apply a good moisturiser to the skin after a shower

Maintenance

- Clean surface area of the chakra therapy table with a disinfectant suitable for ceramic tiles
- Please ensure that the floor is kept clean and dry prior to the guest entering the room

The Use and Application of the Reflexology Basins

By: Jane Crebbin-Bailey HCB Associates

Benefit of treatment

A relaxing effervescent warm foot bath with heated individual seats. This provides a central area for interaction between spa goers and the experiences of the herb bath, laconium, sauna and ice grotto.

Advantages

- Provides a central area for interaction between spa goers and the experiences of the herb bath, laconium, sauna and Ice grotto
- The temperature operates at between 33–38°C
- Fully-tiled and heated seats for 4 persons
- Speed control unit
- Air blower

Contra-indications and precautions

- Skin diseases, such as severe eczema or open psoriasis
- Client feels unwell with a fever
- Infected skin wounds
- Foot infections
- Uncontrolled epilepsy

Preparation

- Operator/reception – First part of the day – Turn on the system as per manufacturer's instructions (see 'Daily Operating Instructions Card')
- Ensure that the area is clean and dry

Method

The reflexology basins should be included as part of a sequence:

- Guests leave the reflexology basins to rest in the relaxation area or meditation room or continue on with another spa experience
- Relax on your towel on the heated ceramic benches and place feet into the bath
- Press the button in front of you
- The water reaches a certain level and stops filling
- This activates the water jets in the base of the basin
- Duration of 5 minutes
- The water automatically drains and then rinses with disinfectant. *NB The water will also drain if you remove your feet from the basin*
- Return to another spa experience involved in a sequence

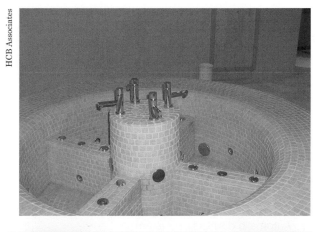

HCB Associates

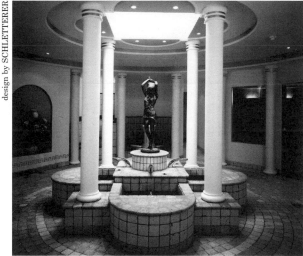

design by SCHLETTERER

www.thermarium.com

After care

- Rest for about 20 minutes, preferably in a warm gown on a recliner
- Drink several glasses of water
- Apply a good moisturiser to the skin after a shower

Maintenance

- Read 'Daily Operating Instructions Card'
- Clean the reflexology basins with a disinfectant suitable for ceramic tiles
- Please ensure that the floor is kept clean and dry surrounding the reflexology basins
- Check cleanliness of area on a regular basis – towels, floor area, etc.

www.spa-therapy.com

The Use and Application of the Thermarium Cleopatra Slipper Bath

By: Jane Crebbin-Bailey HCB Associates

Benefit of the Cleopatra slipper bath

This spa experience promotes relaxation as it soothes away minor aches and pains, releasing tension and stress. The client feels healthier, invigorated and more energetic. The Cleopatra slipper pool is a relaxing hydro jet bath in a sensory haven of milk and aromatics, music and soft light to create an Egyptian experience.

Advantages

- Automatic water massage
- Fits the shape of the body
- Computer controlled for accuracy of temperature and method of application
- Precisely timed sequences and programmes
- Automatic filling and emptying
- Automatic disinfection system

Contra-indications

- Pregnancy (not in the first three months)
- Menstruation
- Cardiovascular disease (severe heart failure, coronary disease, recent stroke or uncontrolled angina)
- Low/high blood pressure
- Skin diseases, such as severe eczema or open psoriasis
- Infected skin wounds
- Severe varicose veins (avoid the lower limb jets)
- Respiratory disease – severe asthma requiring regular inhaler use
- Uncontrolled epilepsy
- Unwell with a fever/vomiting/diarrhoea
- Diabetes

Preparation

- Show the bath to the client prior to filling it
- Fill the bath to the shoulder line to a maximum temperature of 36°C
- Add appropriate product, *plus* chlorine-based tablet to the water, as the bath is filling at the head end of the bath
- The use of candles or night-lights around the bath enhances the ambience

Product use

- Suitable water-based aromatics/seaweeds/milks

Please check with product manufacturer's guidelines for further contra-indications

Precautions/panic button

- If client feels unwell *DO NOT* help the client out of the bath without first following the correct procedure:

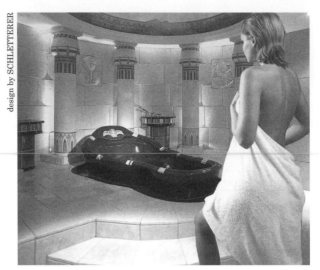

design by SCHLETTERER

www.trofana.at

1. Stop all jets/switches
2. Start to empty the bath – at the same time fill with cold water to decrease the temperature
3. Once the temperature of the water has been lowered just empty it
4. Help the client out of the bath

Method

- It's advisable for the client to take a shower prior to the bath
- Help your client into the bath
- Ensure that the spinal column is centrally placed and aligned to the jets
- Start the bath
- Leave client for maximum 20 minutes, continually checking on his/her comfort

After care

- Rest for about 20 minutes, preferably in a warm gown on a recliner
- Drink several glasses of still water
- Apply a good moisturiser to the skin after a shower

Maintenance of the bath

- Clean bath according to manufacturer's and company guidelines with a suitable proprietary cleaner
- Rinse the bath thoroughly after each client
- Never use anything abrasive on the bath
- Leave the bath clean and dry overnight
- Rinse and clean the bath and jets every morning ready for the first client

The Use and Application of Hydro Pools in Spa treatments

By: Jane Crebbin-Bailey HCB Associates

Benefit of hydrotherapy

Hydrotherapy promotes relaxation as it soothes away minor aches and pains, releasing tension and stress. The client feels healthier, invigorated and more energetic.

Advantages

- Automatic water massage
- Computer controlled for accuracy of temperature and method of application
- Variable applications:
  - specific areas of the body treated by high-pressure jets

Contra-indications and precautions

- Pregnancy (not in the first four months)
- Menstruation/coil – irritable bowl syndrome (DO NOT use the stomach jet)
- Cardiovascular disease (severe heart failure, coronary disease, recent stroke or uncontrolled angina)
- Low blood pressure
- Skin diseases, such as severe eczema or open psoriasis
- Infected skin wounds
- Severe varicose veins (avoid the lower limb jets)
- Respiratory disease – severe asthma requiring regular inhaler use
- Uncontrolled epilepsy
- Unwell with a fever
- Diabetes

Preparation

- Operator/reception – First part of the day – Turn on system as per manufacturer's instructions (see 'Daily Operating Instructions Card')
- Check temperature of water
- Carry out water testing procedure

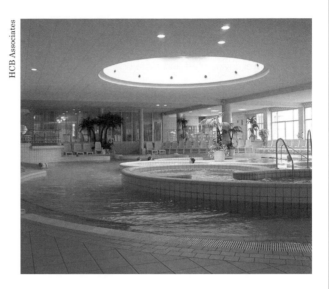

HCB Associates

Method

- It's advisable for the client to take a shower prior to the hydro pool

After care

- Rest for about 20 minutes, preferably in a warm gown on a recliner
- Drink several glasses of still water
- Apply a good moisturiser to the skin after a shower

Maintenance of the Pool

- Read 'Daily Operating Instructions Card'
- Carry out water testing procedure
- Ensure that excess water surrounding the pool on the floor is removed regularly

The Use and Application of Hydrotherapy Baths in Spa Treatments
By: Jane Crebbin-Bailey HCB Associates

Benefit of hydrotherapy

Hydrotherapy promotes relaxation as it soothes away minor aches and pains, releasing tension and stress. The client feels healthier, invigorated and more energetic.

Advantages

- Automatic water massage
- Fits the shape of the body
- Computer controlled for accuracy of temperature and method of application
- Variable applications:
  - specific areas of the body treated by high-pressure jets
  - precise timed sequences and programmes
  - specific reflex regions being subjected to rapid changes in temperature and pressure

Contra-indications

- Pregnancy (not in the first three months)
- Menstruation/coil – irritable bowl syndrome (DO NOT use ventral ramp (stomach jet))
- Cardiovascular disease (severe heart failure, coronary disease, recent stroke or uncontrolled angina)
- Low/high blood pressure
- Skin diseases, such as severe eczema or open psoriasis
- Infected skin wounds
- Severe varicose veins (avoid the lower limb jets)
- Respiratory disease – severe asthma requiring regular inhaler use
- Uncontrolled epilepsy
- Unwell with a fever/vomiting/diarrhoea
- Diabetes

Preparation

- Show the bath to the client prior to filling it
- Look at the client's height and adjust the foot rest accordingly
- Fill the bath to the shoulder line to a maximum temperature of 34°C
- Add appropriate product to the water, as the bath is filling at the head end of the bath
- Turn on the jets to clear any cold water inside the pipes
- Ensure that the direction of jets will commence at the feet – if appropriate to bath

Product use

- Suitable water based aromatics/seaweeds/milks

Please check with product manufacturer's guidelines for further contra-indications

Precautions/Panic button

- If client feels unwell DO NOT help the client out of the bath without first following the correct procedure:
  1. Stop all jets/switches
  2. Start to empty the bath – at the same time fill with cold water to decrease the temperature

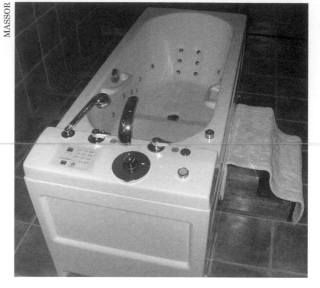

MASSOR

3. Once the temperature of the water has been lowered just empty it
4. Help the client out of the bath

Method

- It's advisable for the client to take a shower prior to the hydrotherapy bath
- Help your client into the bath/make sure that their feet are positioned correctly with the heel on the base of the bath to enable the soles of the feet to be massaged
- Ensure that the spinal column is centrally placed and aligned to the jets
- Start the bath
- Start the direction water jets
- Start the air jets
- Start the programme suitable for your client
- Leave client for maximum 20 minutes, continually checking on his/her comfort

After care

- Rest for about 20 minutes, preferably in a warm gown on a recliner
- Drink several glasses of still water
- Apply a good moisturiser to the skin after a shower

Maintenance of the bath

- Clean bath according to manufacturer's and company guidelines with a suitable proprietary cleaner
- Rinse the bath thoroughly after each client
- Never use anything abrasive on the bath
- Leave the bath clean and dry overnight
- Rinse and clean the bath and jets every morning ready for the first client

The Use and Application of Hydrotherapy Baths in Spa Treatments
By: Jane Crebbin-Bailey HCB Associates

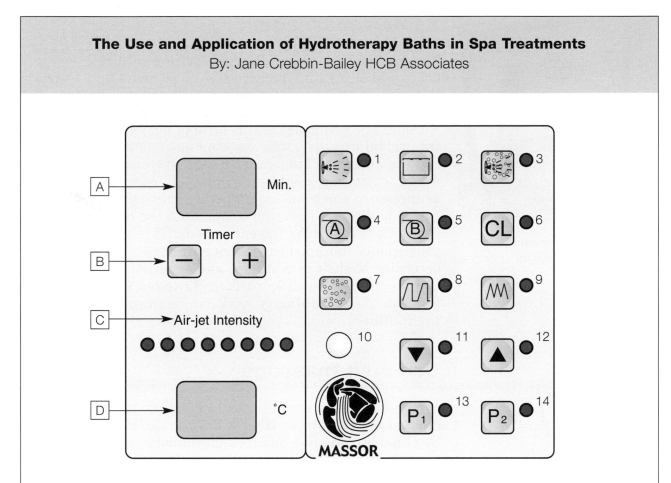

Legend

A.   Water and air timer (in minutes)
B.   Decrease/increase duration of water and air massage
C.   Air massage intensity (bottom of bath) – visual display
D.   Water temperature in bath (°C)

1.   Main water pump
2.   Sequence massage
3.   Air blower through side jets
4.   2nd water pump
5.   Accessory B (100 W Maximum) – optional sub-aqua light/radio
6.   Manual rinsing
7.   Air blower through bottom perforations
8.   Intermittent power variation of air
9.   Continuous power variation of air
10. Infrared receiver (optional)
11. Decrease power of air through bottom perforations
12. Increase power of air through bottom perforations
13. Relaxing programme
14. Stimulating programme

Use of hose for manual lymphatic drainage

Step 1. Stop sequence massage (2) when sequence is at the foot
Step 2. Turn on tap for hose
Step 3. Perform lymphatic drainage massage as shown

www.spa-therapy.com

©HCB Associates – September 2000

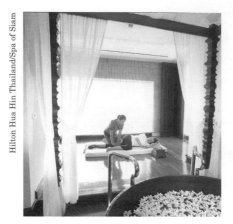

Thai massage, The Spa, Hilton Hotel, Hua Hin, Thailand

Esalen massage

The **Esalen** Institute in Big Sur, California, USA, developed ESALEN®-Bodywork over 30 years ago. Currie Prescott, the director of training at The Centre in Zurich, Switzerland, was the first to bring this bodywork to Europe. The principles of this form of bodywork are traditional massage, long stroking movements, gentle rocking and stretching, passive joint exercise, deep muscle work, sensitive cranial balancing, and precise Chinese acupressure point massage. This therapy is given with a gentle and conscious touch to heighten the body's sensory perceptions and relax the entire body. The practitioner/therapist can develop their own style according to their own studies and experiences, therefore specific methods such as **rolfing**, **Traeger work**, Feldenkrais and **polarity** work can be incorporated into the routine.

Swedish massage

Swedish massage is a traditional massage technique created in 1812 by Per Henrik Ling at the University of Stockholm using five different movements of massage (known as classical movements) resulting in a firm but gentle pressure. It is used to improve the circulation, ease muscle aches and tension, improve flexibility and create relaxation.

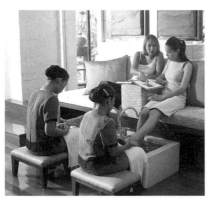

Foot massage at The Spa, Hilton Hotel, Hua Hin, Thailand; Foot massage is very popular in Thailand with shops on every street. It is often given in spas as a ritual prior to a treatment

Hydro massage

Hydro massage is an underwater massage performed in a hydro bath equipped with high pressure jets and a hand manipulated hose to stimulate the blood and lymphatic circulations.

Polarity massage

Polarity massage is a technique created by Dr Randolph Stone of Austria in the 1900s. It involves gently rocking, holding and massaging the body, and is designed to balance the body's subtle or electromagnetic energy. A four-part programme is developed to restore the body's correct energy balance using touch, stretching exercises, diet and mental-emotional balanced attitude.

Lomi lomi

The word *lomi* comes from the Hawaiian language, meaning massage, and working the inner and outer of the body. Duplicating the word **lomi lomi**, intensifies its meaning, making it important massage. This holistic treatment, using a lot of warmed oil, unleashes tension in the body as well as treating the five senses with music and touch.

Stone therapy

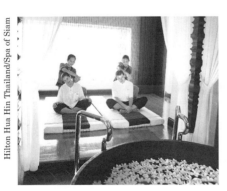

Stone therapy

Stone therapy is based on American Indian folklore and therapy. It utilizes ancient volcanic stones from the Arizona Desert, which have been moulded and shaped by time from water and sand. Some of the stones are heated and others are frozen to provide a very deep massage. The client lies back on the heated stones that have been carefully placed under the back, others are placed between the toes and fingers and on the chakra points, aromatic oils are then applied. The client is massaged with the hot or the cold stones to stimulate or relax them, working with the flow of energy in order to balance the chakras.

Shiatsu

SHI, meaning finger, and ATSU, meaning pressure, form the word shiatsu. This massage technique was developed in Japan by Tokujiro Namikoshi in the 1940s. It works the energy meridians to stimulate the body's inner powers of balance and healing using pressure from the fingers, palms, elbows, knees or feet. Shiatsu corrects and maintains the proper position of the bones, the muscles and the meridians to balance the body's energy (*chi*) and nervous system. Shiatsu is performed on the floor on a mat and the guest wears light cotton clothes.

Indian head massage

Indian head massage, The Spa, Hilton Hotel, Hua Hin, Thailand

This is a relaxing head and scalp massage, traditionally given by mothers to their children in India. In Hindi 'champi' is the word used for head massage. It is a combination of acupressure and shiatsu movements on the head, scalp, shoulders, upper back, arms and hands that releases tension, stimulates the blood and lymph circulations and rebalances energy.

Envelopment treatments

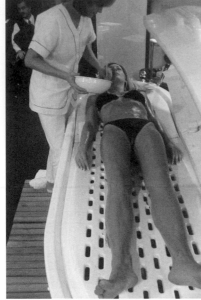

Seaweed Envelopment

There is a range of envelopment treatments in which, as the name suggests, the body is cocooned in a blanket, electric blanket, linen wraps, sand (Psamo), sheets, towels, **seaweed wrap** or in a Soft Pack, Dry Float treatment bed or steam cabinet machine. Products are applied to the body and the client relaxes for approximately 20 minutes whilst the products are absorbed in through the skin.

Balinese Boreh

Boreh is an ancient Balinese spice body mask made from a mixture of indigenous herbs and spices, including ginger, cloves, nutmeg, cinnamon, pepper, Javanese long pepper, *Curcuma heyneana* (turmeric), and rice powder to create a treatment to warm the body.

Javanese lulur

Lulur comes from the Javanese language of Indonesia, meaning 'coating the skin' and traditionally a treatment for a bride prior to her wedding, and has been practised in the palaces of Java since the seventeenth century. It is a body scrub and skin polishing treatment that uses a mixture of finely ground herbs, spices and the roots of plants indigenous to Java, Indonesia. Fenugreek, turmeric, sandalwood and rice powder are mixed to a paste with Jasmine oil, that is applied to the body to dry and then rubbed off. Yoghurt is then applied as its lactic acid, softens the skin. The final part of the treatment is a fragrant flower filled bath of rose, jasmine, ylang ylang or frangipani.

Sound therapy

Sound therapy refers to a range of therapies in which sound is used to treat the body both physically and mentally. A synthesis of sounds and techniques have been used around the world since ancient times to aid healing, as part of religious occasions or to toll an event. In 1896 American physicians discovered that certain music improved the thought processes and increased blood circulation. Music therapy was used during the Second World War as a part of a rehabilitation programme for soldiers. In Europe, in the 1950s and 1960s, sound wave machines were developed.

Treatment by sound waves is thought to bring balance and harmony to the body and be performed through the use of musical instruments, chanting or voice.

The British osteopath Peter Manners developed a sound wave machine to deliver treatments using healing vibrations; a process known as **cymatics** or cymatic medicine. The machine uses a frequency that is set to match the same frequency of the healthy cells, thereby making the cells vibrate at a healthy resonance. Cymatics has been used in the treatment of cancer. Manners went on to develop a computerised system with about 800 frequencies. This system is sometimes known as bioresonance or vibrational therapy.

Dr Alfred Tomatis and Dr Guy Berard, two ear specialists from France, developed a therapy called the **Tomatis method** of 'auditory integration training'. This involves listening to sounds through headphones and is used to treat a variety of conditions from dyslexia, anxiety, chronic fatigue syndrome, autism, pain and behavioural problems.

Chanting and toning can allow the body to reach a meditative state by producing the pure sound of a drawn out vowel and is believed to release emotions like stress or pain and produce a state of well-being. In Tibet monks use bronze singing bowls in conjunction with chanting.

Transpersonal Soundtherapy®

Dr Wolfgang Koelbl and his wife, Dr Ruth Koelbl, have created an energy medicine treatment method known as Transpersonal Soundtherapy®. This works on the body and spirit, primarily on the emotions and thoughts by looking at how breathing rhythms and the pulse rate can work with the chakras (energy centres of the body), endogenous vibrations, energy meridians and tension in the muscles. It seeks to activate the chakras. Vibrations are not only heard, but are picked up by the whole body.

Transpersonal Soundtherapy® works at a deep level of consciousness – that of deep relaxation or trance. Different tone vibrations and frequencies are created a variety of instruments and sound tools. The effect of music and sound is to increase the neuronal networks in the brain, maximising the creativity of the brain's performance. The music, say Drs Koelbl, corresponds in the human perception to a journey through consciousness at deeper levels, where the sound experience starts to create pictures and the brain tries to interpret the 'heard' sound experience. This sound therapy is 'a universal language which can be understood directly by the emotions and the soul, without restriction

Fascinating Fact

Fabien Maman, French sound healer has written a book entitled *The Role of Music in the 21st Century*.

A musical instrument called the 'Pythagorean tone generator' produces unique sounds that correspond to the chakras of the body. Each note produced from the Pythagorean scale (Pythagorus 569 BC, Greek philosopher and mathematician) are said to balance and cleanse the chakras creating harmony from chaos and when seen on an oscilloscope (instrument showing sound waves) each note is a perfect circle.

The unique sounds correspond to the chakra, for example the base chakra corresponds to 'C' the 1st position and the throat chakra 'G' corresponds to the 5th position. The perfect musical 5th (C to G) contain all the tones of creation, the 'OM', the sound of the Universe.

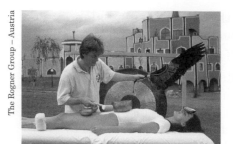

Dr Wolgang Koelbl practising sound therapy at The Rogner Bad Blumau Spa in Austria

from intellectual patterns and beliefs. The human being can be immediately touched and reconnected with experiences in a new and loving way, resulting in a form of reincarnation or reintegration therapy.'

Some of the instruments used in this energy therapy are: a Monochord, a sound-vibration bed, Tibetan singing bowls, gongs, tam tams, tubular bells of all sizes and of different tones, Circle of the fifth by Maman in order to activate the chakras, a sound pyramid (whose measurements are proportional to those of the Cheops pyramid and covered with tubular bells), quartz bowls, ocean drum, water phone, rattles, bells, drums, plants and big feathers. To receive the benefit of this therapy, clients must experience three phases:

1. *first phase* – introduction to a deep relaxation and trance state of mind

2. *second phase* – consciousness journey, conscious dreams

3. *third phase* – the cautious return to reality.

Many people experience an increase in energy and in addition to seeing inner pictures, colours and abstract feelings, the whole body is better balanced and feels more in harmony with itself. Many have testified that it is a unique experience.

Colour therapy

Fascinating Fact

Dowsing charts – method of measuring a physical state with a selected 'dowsing tool', for example a pendulum

Colour is another form of energy medicine (see page 139). Colours have energies and vibrate at a specific frequency. Though it is an age-old treatment, colour therapy was re-invented in the 1950s by Theo Gimbel, who based his ideas on old mystical texts and asserted that matter could be considered as 'solidified Light'. The body is thought to respond to light at different wavelengths and each individual possesses a personal wavelength to which he or she responds more readily than to others. Like sound therapy, the use of colour therapy is said to enhance positive energies.

Many therapists believe in the Vedic theory of the body's chakras and try to discover which colours are missing and need be replaced to keep the chakras balanced and working in harmony. This is done using 'dowsing' charts of the spine that correspond to various colours and body areas, or by colour reflection readings from eight coloured charts from which the client makes choices.

Treatment may consist of colour illumination therapy where the person, clothed in white, is bathed in the colour required to balance the chakras or replace the missing colour. The primary colour is alternated for a set time with its complementary colour. The use of complementary colours is said to ensure a healthy balance in the body. Clients may also be asked to wear 'their' colours. Colour therapy is used to treat a variety of conditions from addiction and depression to fatigue, insomnia and nervous tension.

The Ancient Egyptians built temples of healing with colour, to worship the sun god, Re, the god of light. The Pharaohs prayed each morning to the god Re for energy and to revitalise the spirit. They used many natural plants to obtain the colours needed for their paintings on the walls and floors of temples and pyramids. They painted green on the floor and blue on the ceilings – the colours of grass and sky – to emulate nature.

The Greek physician Hippocrates considered colour to be a science. During the Middle Ages, Paracelsus (1493–1541), a Swiss physician and alchemist, reintroduced the knowledge of the Ancient Egyptians and practised healing with colour, herbs and music.

The scientist, Isaac Newton, wrote about the relationship between light and energy (*Optics*, published in 1704). He discovered the reflection of light through a prism and saw the seven colours of the spectrum that can be seen in the rainbow – red, orange, yellow, green, blue, indigo and violet.

Albert Szent-Gyorgi, a Nobel Prize winner, discovered Vitamin C by studying the effects of photosynthesis. He came to realise that the sun's energy is stored in plants and believed that this energy could be passed on to us and other living creatures.

Colours have energies (an electromagnetic field) and vibrate at a specific frequency. Light is absorbed through our eyes and skin. We need a minimum of 20 minutes of the sun's ultraviolet rays to activate a form of cholesterol, which is present in the skin, to convert it to Vitamin D. A well-known effect of light deficiency is Seasonal Affective Disorder (SAD), causing depression related disorders.

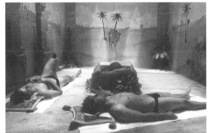

SAD (Seasonal Affective Disorder) Therapy in a relaxarium by Haslauer GmbH, Austria

Fascinating Fact

Vitamin D aids in the absorption of calcium from the intestinal tract and the breakdown of the assimilation of phosphorus that is necessary for the formation of bones. A deficiency of this vitamin leads to rickets, poorly developed muscles, nervous irritability and a retention of phosphorus in the kidney.

Aura-Soma

Aura-Soma, another form of colour therapy, is a 'non-invasive self-selective soul therapy', according to its creator, Vicky Wall, a blind chiropodist. Aura-Soma, uses a system of colour therapy that has been created from the living energies of plants, minerals and light. Liquid colours are made by combining vegetable oil and water that have been subjected to the energies of crystals and gems and the energies of light and colour.

A choice of four colour combinations is made up from 90 'balance' bottles, containing two coloured liquids, a mixture of essential oils on a layer of spring water containing a herbal mixture. The colours chosen are said to provide insight into the emotional and physical condition of the one seeking help. The meaning of the 'chosen' colours is interpreted by the therapist. The contents of the shaken bottles are applied to the skin daily for as long as necessary. Aura-Soma is used to treat chronic emotional and stress-related conditions.

Colour energised water

Colour energised water treatments have been used since the Ancient Egyptians and also in Ayurvedic medicine. Coloured glass bottles, vases or jars are filled with water, gemstones are sometimes placed in the container and then the liquid is placed in direct sunlight to colour-solarise the contents. This method is used for milk in Ayurvedic medicine. The different colours are thought to have either a sedating, energising, cooling, antiseptic or cleansing effect. The use of aromatics and coloured water in the bath is an alternative form of colour therapy.

Crystals and gemstones are another use of colour and energy for healing. The stones are placed either around or on the meridian points of the body, in the home, office, on VDUs and other electrical equipment to absorb bad vibrations and positive ions. It is considered that gemstones absorb and retain electromagnetic vibrations that are released with different effects. For instance, crystals can stimulate energy and protect the body; wearing amethyst on the chest is said to help someone who suffers with bronchitis.

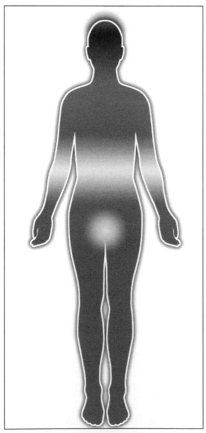

Aura-Soma Products Ltd

The chakras

The chakra, from the Sanskrit meaning 'wheel', represents the seven colours of the spectrum and the four elements — earth, fire, water and air. The chakra centres are situated along the spine (*sushumna*) and connected via our energy channels or meridians (*nadis*) to the organs of the body. Each of the 72,000 nadis criss-cross the chakra distributing energy (*chi* or *prana*) to each major nerve or glandular centre in the body. When one chakra is out of balance, others become affected.

Red   The base chakra (the mudlahara – root)

Gemstone   *Ruby*
Planet   *The sun*

Red, the root chakra, represents our foundation and survival. This is the first energy centre and is located at the base of the spine. It relates to earth and keeps you grounded.

The red chakra is physical vitality; it stimulates the blood circulation, combats negative thoughts and emotions. Although a warm and sensual colour, too much red is said to trigger anger, irritability and impatience. This colour is often associated with 'fast food' chains.

The secondary colour to red is pink, considered emotionally soothing, nurturing and surrounding us with love and protection. As an experiment in the UK, some prisons walls have been painted pink, as it is thought to lessen irritation and aggression. It is reported to have had a marked improvement on prisoners' behaviour.

Orange   The small of the back – spleen centre

Orange is a joyous, uplifting colour and represents the freedom of feelings and emotions. It relates to the navel area, abdomen, sex organs and periphery of the body. Orange stimulates the mind and alleviates feelings of self-pity.

The secondary colour to orange is peach or apricot for laughter, creativity, independence and security.

Yellow   The middle of the back – solar plexus centre

Gemstone   *Yellow sapphire*
Planet   *Jupiter*

Yellow is a happy, bright uplifting colour and represents the intellectual side of the brain and the ability to express oneself. It is good for the memory and decision making as well as the assimilation of ideas and it encourages an optimistic attitude. It relates to the solar plexus area.

The secondary colour to yellow is dull yellow/mustard – the colour of fear.

Green   The centre of the shoulder blades – heart centre

Gemstone   *Emerald*
Planet   *Mercury*

Green is the colour of relaxation and has an earthy, natural feel to it like the colour of grass, it represents physical and emotional balance.

Green relates to the chest and heart area and regulates circulation. This is the colour of Islam and also of Tara, one of the goddess manifestations of Buddha.

The secondary colour, olive green, suggests decay and is considered to be negative. Lime green relates to the emotions of envy and resentment.

Blue   Base of the skull – the throat centre and thyroid

Gemstone   *Blue sapphire*
Planet   *Saturn*

Blue, like the sky and the sea, is a cool, calming peaceful colour that represents the higher part of the mind, inspiring clarity and control of the mind. Blue is the colour of a member of a Hindu high caste and of aristocratic Krishna; it is associated with the life-giving monsoons. It relates to the throat area and communication. Blue helps to lower blood pressure.

The secondary colours of blue are dark blue, midnight blue and turquoise. Dark blue is thought to be effective in pain relief; midnight blue connects us to the feminine and intuitive side of our brain and turquoise, heightens sensitivity, creativity and communication. Turquoise also alleviates tiredness and mental strain and helps to fight infections.

Indigo   The Brow centre – the third eye and pineal gland

Indigo is a mystical colour that stimulates imagination and creativity. It represents the third eye and is one of the major chakras associated with psychic abilities, intuition, spiritualism and clairvoyance. It is said to combat shock and fear, to cleanse emotions and to repel mosquitoes, it is a protective colour. Too much indigo has narcotic properties.

Violet/purple   The crown centre and pituitary gland

Violet is an inspiring colour that represents spirituality. It balances the metabolism and suppresses hunger. Violet is cooling for sunburn and heat rash.

Magenta   Above the head – etheric

Magenta is an uplifting and spiritual colour that represents compassion, support and kindness.

White

White is at the centre of all colours.

Meditation

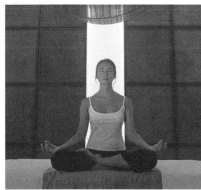

Mediation at The Spa, Hilton Hotel, Hua Hin, Thailand

Meditation is not a religion, although it is often central to the practice of different religions, Buddhism for example. It is advisable to begin training with an experienced teacher either in a group or one to one. Many doctors recognise that the physiological benefits of meditation help to reduce stress, lower blood pressure, reduce muscular aches and pains and help asthma sufferers. More alpha waves are produced in the brain during meditation, allowing the body and mind to relax but maintain a receptive state that increases mental clarity.

The objective of meditation is to focus the mind, to free it of thoughts, without dwelling on the purpose or reason, to achieve *Nirvana* – enlightenment. This can be done through various techniques, and it's important to find one you are comfortable working with: The most famous symbolic picture is the **Wheel of Sri**, known as 'sri yantra'. Yantras, or **mandalas**, originate in the Eastern religions, such as Buddhism, and are usually geometric shapes intended to focus the mind.

Visualisation

Visualisation involves either looking at an object such as a flower, stone, burning candle or patch on the wall and then visualising it in your mind or using your visual imagination to create pictures in your mind.

Koans

These are questions set by a Zen Buddhist master to consider 'what is the sound of one hand clapping?', 'what is infinity?', or, 'what is nothing?'. These thoughts are to be considered through intuition rather then by logical processes.

Mantras

A sound, phrase, sacred word or syllable, used as an object of concentration and chanted aloud or silently to oneself. The word mantra is from the Sanskrit *man* – to think. Perhaps the most well-known mantra of compassion is 'Om Mani Padme Hum'. *Om* is considered by the Hindu's to be the sound of the vibration of the universe. 'Alleluia' is an equivalent Christian mantra.

Transcendental meditation

Known as TM, this technique is based upon Hindu traditions, originated by Maharishi Majesh Yogi, an Indian monk, for relaxing and creating awareness in the mind and body through the silent repetition of a mantra. Thoughts are said to transcend to a deeper state of consciousness to bring about tranquillity and creativity.

Yoga

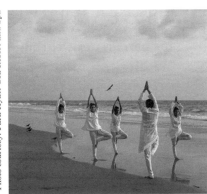

Photo courtesy: Park Hyatt Goa Resort and Spa

Yoga

Yoga is a Hindu discipline from the ancient Vedic civilisation of India (2800 BCE, Before Christian Era) composed of five principles – focused deep breathing (Pranayama), stretching and toning the body using various positions designed to improve circulation, flexibility and strength (Asanas), nutrition, meditation and relaxation. Yoga is a philosophical approach to balancing the body and mind. Many teachers of yoga have since developed their own variations that are practised today. One example is given below.

Ashtanga yoga

Based upon the teachings of a guru called Sri T. Krishnamacharya, Ashtanga yoga is a unique form of Hatha (physical) yoga using vinyasas – breath-synchronised movements.

Oxygen therapy

Oxygen is an element. It has the atomic number 8 and an atomic weight of 15.9994, a melting point of −218.4°C (−361.1°F), a boiling point of −183.0°C (−297.4°F), a density of 1.429g/1 (1atm, 0°C), and a Valence of 2–6 or $1s^2 2s^2 2p4$. Pure oxygen is 1.1 times heavier than air.

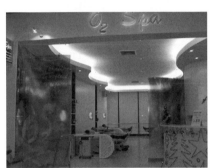

Oxygen Therapy, Spa Ozone, Bangkok airport, Thailand

Emotional stress uses the body's oxygen reserves to produce more adrenaline-related hormones. The stress of modern day living robs the body of oxygen to neutralise excess acidity. This lack of oxygen is said to account for anger and behaviour-related problems.

Oxygen therapy – ozone therapy, hyperbaric chambers (operating at pressures higher than normal) – may reverse this action by allowing the blood to absorb more oxygen, and therefore nutrients into the body's system, resulting in an increase of energy and well-being. The benefits are reported to improve memory, micro-circulatory conditions, exhaustion, metabolic problems and energy and to stimulate the immune system.

Fascinating Fact

On Earth, in the upper atmosphere, the gaseous oxygen is called triatomic oxygen O^3 ozone and monatomic oxygen O. In the lower atmosphere, oxygen consists of molecules of 2 atoms, O^2.

Ozone, from the Greek word, meaning 'smell' (O^3), is found in the stratosphere where it is referred to as the 'ozone layer'. It plays an important role by absorbing the harmful ultraviolet rays of the sun and thereby protecting Earth.

The carbon dioxide (CO^2) bath

Carbon dioxide baths are popular in Europe. The gas is used in two ways – either in a plastic body bag closed at the waist or neck, or by saturating a saline solution with the gas at normal barometric pressure and a temperature of 33°C. The gas is absorbed through the skin, causing dilation of the blood vessels and increasing the circulation; the client feels warm and well. These baths are also used to relieve pain, and contractures in scars. A drop in systolic blood pressure of up to 5mm of mercury and a sense of euphoria have also been observed.

Ayurveda

Ayurveda is a Sanskrit word derived from *ayur* (life) and *veda* (knowledge). It has come to mean the science of life and it encompasses the body, mind and spirit. This ancient form of medicine has been in continuous practice for more than 5000 years. It is a holistic approach to health that balances the body, mind and consciousness.

Sanskrit is an ancient language of India, of the Vedas, Hinduism, and of philosophical and scientific literature. It is the oldest recorded member of the Indo-European family of languages (Greek and Latin). It is one of the official languages of India, but is only used for religious purposes.

It takes four years to study and become an Ayurvedic physician, learning traditional Ayurvedic procedures for purification and rejuvenation, which include oil massage, acupressure massage, herbal steam treatment, shirodhama, Gregorian and Vedic chants, classical and modern Gandharva Veda, cleansing diet, herbal therapy, nutrition, yoga, Jyotish (Vedic astrology), Sanskrit and lifestyle education.

The philosophies of Ayurveda take into account the natural elements of air, earth, water, fire and space (space is all-inclusive – consciousness and internal space), as well as *prana* – life force or energy. The structure of the body is made up of the 'elements' and the functions (constitution) of the body are governed by the three **doshas**:

1. *Vata* (air) thin or underweight. Physical conditions – dry skin, constipation. Mental conditions – nervous disposition. Creative, balanced and adaptable.

2. *Pitta* (fire) excess heat. Physical conditions – heat related disorders. Mental conditions – hot tempered, irritable. Good leaders, warm and goal orientated.

3. *Kapha* (water) excess water. Physical conditions – congestion, overweight. Mental conditions – lethargy, indulgent. Strong, muscular, calm and loyal.

According to Ayurveda, there are seven body types:

1. *Mono types* – vata, pitta or kapha predominant.

2. *Dual types* – vata–pitta, pitta–kapha or kapha–vata.

3. *One equal type* – vata, pitta and kapha in equal proportions.

Every individual has a combination of these three doshas and to understand individuality is the foundation of healing.

Ayurveda offers therapies for each of the five senses:

1. *taste* – herbs and nutrition

2. *touch* – massage (abhyanga), yoga and exercise

3. *smell* – aromatherapy

4. *sight* – colour therapy

5. *hearing* – sound therapy.

It is considered that the sixth sense is spirituality, manifesting as mantra meditation, chanting and living ethically.

Many Ayurveda treatments have been developed; the following are a sample of the body massage therapies.

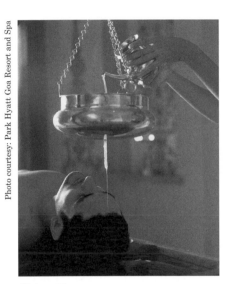

Shirodhara

Abhyanga – massage

There are three types of abhyanga: vata, pitta and kapha, which vary in depth, speed and sequence of stroke. A relaxing application of oil is used to stimulate and increase circulation.

- *Pinda abhyanga* – this massage incorporates the same techniques as abhyanga and uses a mixture of herbal milk and rice, to feed and nurture the skin.
- *Vishesh* – a firm pressured massage with a squeezing action that helps to eliminate deeply rooted toxins.
- *Shirodhara* – massage combined with a heat treatment; steam oil is poured over the forehead to a particular pattern and temperature. A profoundly relaxing treatment that balances the nervous system, producing a quiet meditative state.
- *Shiro **Basti*** – an ancient, soothing Vedic therapy said to help headaches and memory loss. A container (similar to a hat) is placed on the head whereupon warm herbal oil is poured into the container and left for 20 minutes to absorb into the scalp.

Source: The Ayurvedic Institute. Dr. Lad, Pune, Mumbai, India.

F.X. Mayr Cure

Dr Franz Xavier Mayr (1875–1965) was an Austrian physician who founded the Mayr Diagnostic Method, Mayr Therapy and the famous Mayr® Cure. As a medical student, he became interested in the characteristics of a healthy intestinal tract and stomach, and realised that there was no diagnostic criterion differentiating between a healthy and impaired digestive system, he developed a treatment that comprised a special diet and intestinal cleansing. Mayr recognised that continuous excessive demands on the

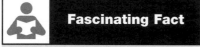

digestive organs resulted in insufficient production and quantity of the digestive juices, creating poor absorption of nutrients.

The Mayr Cure is an intensive intestinal detoxification and cleansing programme in consultation with a doctor, resulting in improved digestion, metabolism, energy and well-being. The three principles of the Mayr Cure are:

1. conservation
2. cleansing
3. learning.

Conservation

The doctor will advise on the correct diet from tea fasting to milk and bread, progressing to special detoxifying diets and spa cuisine.

Cleansing

Cleansing the digestive tract includes de-acidification of the connective tissues, muscles, and organs of the body. Palatable salt (Epsom salts) and thermal water are taken as a part of the cleansing drinking treatment. Physical and manual (abdominal) treatments support the cleansing programme.

Learning

This element looks at the function and the biorhythms of the body. It includes learning how to eat and chew the food correctly.

The Mayr treatment programme is suitable for the following conditions:

- digestive disturbances – diarrhoea, constipation, candida, acidity
- stress related and psychosomatic disorders
- migraines and headaches
- skin allergies and diseases
- weak immune system
- lower back pain
- arthritis, rheumatism, and gout
- obesity, circulatory, cardiovascular and blood pressure disorders.

A full treatment programme lasts for four weeks.

Product use

Life is experienced through our senses. The use of products not only facilitates a treatment but should stimulate the five senses.

Sight

Certain products are coloured, which is pleasing to the eye. Colour can have a powerful effect on how we feel – hence colour therapy – light stimulates the body's endocrine system and energy centres.

Taste

A glass of water prior to a treatment has a diuretic effect and helps relieve fluid retention problems.

Smell

The use of essential oils and/or seaweed in the bath or treatments stimulates the olfactory receptors.

Touch

The care of the therapist whilst giving a treatment provides comfort. This aspect of therapy includes the touch of the fabrics against the skin and the way a client/guest is greeted.

Hearing

Music helps to release tension and stress and can be uplifting or meditative. Sophrology is a method of relaxation using low frequency sound that lowers the pulse rate.

Essential oils

Essential oils are highly concentrated, very volatile organic oils present in various plants, usually containing **terpenes** and **esters** and the odour or flavour from the plant of which they are an extract. Oleoresin is a semi-solid mixture of a resin and an essential oil, obtained from certain plants. Whereas a fixed oil is a natural animal or vegetable oil that is not volatile, an oleoresin is a mixture of esters and fatty acids, usually triglycerides.

Distillation uses water or steam to remove oils from dried or fresh plants, leaves, bark or roots. Other methods of extraction include cold pressing, alcohol or solvents. Lavender is one of the easiest plants from which to make an extraction. It takes approximately 100 kilos of lavender to produce one litre of essential oil. Essential oils are absorbed through the skin and into the blood stream. To be used safely, they should be used with a carrier oil or water, as essential oils can cause skin irritation or allergic reactions.

The Greeks, Egyptians, Indians and Romans used essential oils as perfume, for massage and for trade. They have been found in 3000-year-old tombs of Egyptian pharaohs and high priestesses. The physician Hippocrates refers to essential oils for their healing, massage and psychological benefits, as did Galen. As long as 5000 years ago, the ancient civilisations of Mesopotamia had equipment for extracting essential oils from plants. Ayurvedic medicine, cherished by the ancient Vedic civilisations of India, advocated the use of an essential oil massage as a part of their holistic teachings.

Aromatics or micro-emulsions bring all the benefits of natural plant extracts to give soothing, relaxing, de-stressing, detoxifying, stimulating and hydrating effects to enhance the benefits of the treatment. Herbs or flowers can be put in a muslin bag and tied then put into a bath to give a wonderful scent and powerful infusion to the water; for example, lavender, rosemary or jasmine flowers, rose petals or peppermint leaves. Similarly, herbs or flowers can be tied in a posy and placed on the treatment couch or pillow to have a visual effect as well as to scent the air. Aromatic candles and burners, pot pourri, bath and body products with added essential oils can be found everywhere.

Milk baths/whey and oil-cream baths

Milk baths are rich in calcium, potassium, sodium and magnesium and also contain vitamins A, B, C and D. Cleopatra was said to have bathed in a bath of asses' milk and whey (rich in linoleic acid), olive oil and honey, which benefits a dry, stressed or sensitive skin. Today it is possible to recreate the same luxurious sensation with the addition of jasmine flowers and rose petals.

Kurland goat butter has anti-inflammatory properties ideal for neurodermatitis, eczema, psoriasis or rheumatic complaints of the joints. Evening primrose oil or cream bath is used as a dermatological treatment for early ageing, neurodermatitis and psoriasis.

Coconut

Fresh or dried coconut is rich in vitamins and has cleansing and moisturising properties that can be utilised in exotic treatments when mixed with oils, herbs and flowers, either as body scrubs or in massage therapies.

Sea salts

To create a sense of thalassotherapy in the bath, sea salts not only remineralise the body but the trace elements will give a feeling of well-being and equilibrium.

Seaweeds

Three-quarters of the earth's surface is sea, a vast source of life. Seaweeds capture the natural richness of the sea – trace elements, minerals, amino acids, proteins, etc., which are essential to the human organism.

There are around 25 000 varieties of seaweed recorded. Most of these have therapeutic value. Seaweed is grouped by its colour:

1. cyanophyta – blue seaweeds
2. rhodophyta – red seaweeds
3. phaeophyta – brown seaweeds
4. chlorophyta – green seaweeds.

By adding seaweed products to baths, concentrations of minerals and trace elements are released into the water and absorbed into the body through osmosis, bringing beneficial effects. Seaweed products are either added to the bath or applied to the body, as in a body envelopment treatment.

Laminaria digitata algae (rich in iodine) are found in particularly deep water and are gathered by boat. *Fucus vesiculosis* and *Ascophyllum nodosum* algae grow on rocks and are gathered by fishermen on foot and cut with a sickle. *Spirulina* a blue-green, spiral shaped algae, is rich in protein and vitamin C and found in salt water lakes.

All of these plants have specialised adaptations that protect them against drying when they are exposed during low tide. Most types of kelp are edible and extracts of kelp are used in the manufacture of ice cream and cosmetics. Many companies use seaweed in their face, body and bath products as well as in dietary supplements.

Fascinating Fact

Polyphenols found in seaweed protect it from the sun in a similar way to melanin in the skin of a human being. Look at the seaweed washed up on the beach or rocks and you can see pigmentation marks where it has been exposed to the sun.

Fascinating Fact

The Varbergs Kurort and Kusthotell in Sweden is a conference hotel and thalassotherapy resort, where they offer a treatment using seawater and seaweed. It commences with a relaxing bath of *Laminaria digitata* in a specially designed wooden bathtub. After 10 minutes, the therapist massages the guest with the fresh seaweed, leaving the skin extremely soft.

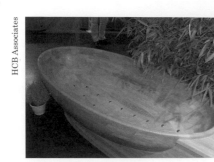

Wooden hydro bath

Fascinating Fact

The main sources of injury to the **thallus** of seaweeds are herbivores, sand abrasion and the force of waves. However, in coenocytic and multi-cellular seaweeds regrowth generally occurs. In multi-cellular seaweeds (i.e. *Fucus vesiculocus*) the sealing of the wound involves changes in the cells or cellular wall formation. In some seaweeds, a newly synthesised sulphated polysaccharide is produced to fill the wound. Some algae chemically defend themselves against herbivore attack and microbial invasion. At a biochemical level, they can produce and distribute polymeric material to allow a rapid 'plugging' of the wound and repair the cell wall. Various families of algae have different processes for this and have the ability to mix two components together – similar to epoxy glue or polyurethane foam.

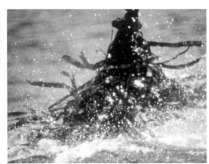

Seaweed Laminaria being harvested from the sea in Brittany

Future products from algae may include methane, alcohols, fatty acids and esters. In the USA there is interest in obtaining energy from seaweeds. Seaweed mariculture involves large-scale cultivation of algae in the sea or in tanks on land. The major seaweed farming countries are Japan, Korea, the Philippines, Indonesia and China, where seaweed with its rich source of vitamins and minerals is grown for food. Agars and carrageenans are produced from red algae and alginates from brown. The two most economically cultivated edible seaweeds are undaria, from Korea, and laminaria, mainly from China; they are dried and eaten in soups, salads, seasonings and tea.

Micronised marine algae have been processed for over 30 years and this is the preferred method adopted by the French company Thalgo, where the cells of the algae are literally exploded to liberate their contents. Conventional processes pulverise and flatten the cells trapping the cellular mass. Micronisation yields a total suspension of the algae and their mineral salts and trace elements in water. The suspension is dried to produce a highly concentrated powder equivalent to over 15 times its weight in fresh plant material. Three types of algae (*Lithothamnium*, *Laminaria digitata*, *Fucus vesiculosis*) are harvested in the North Sea during the equinox when their mineral and trace element concentration is at its maximum. Manufactured in this way, the fine grains of the algae are capable of crossing the skin barrier during an application or hot bath.

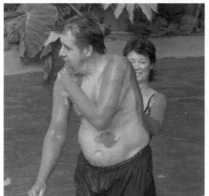

Mud therapy, Glen Ivy Hot
Springs, California, USA

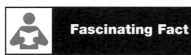

Fascinating Fact

As a natural therapy,
thermal applications of
different kinds of mud
were practised in ancient
times. The famous Greek
physician, Galen, codified
the great benefit given by
these treatments,
particularly in cases of
chronic inflammatory
diseases, arthritis and
rheumatism. Plinius
(23–79 AD) mentioned in
his writings the use of the
Fango mud from the
thermal ponds of Battaglia
near Padua in North Italy.

Mud

Mud is very beneficial in both beauty and medical
treatments. Coastal mud, clay, loam and mud from inland
lakes and peat are used for packs. The name given to this
group, which includes chalk, is Peloids (from the Greek
Pelos), and the therapy is known as **pelotherapy**.

The thermophysical properties of mud and peat largely
depend upon the type being used. Generally, mud is applied
to a particular area of the body, for example the knees,
shoulders, back, hips, etc. for 20 minutes. Muds have
exfoliating properties, increase skin circulation and aid the
removal of waste products.

Parafango mud

Parafango is a dried thermal mud mixed with paraffin (to
make it more malleable), talcum and magnesium oxide to
prevent precipitation. The pack is completely dehydrated
and the heat exchange is produced via conduction.
Parafango packs are applied at a higher temperature –
50°C (122°F) than hydrated peloids, which are used at 45°C
(113°F). There is a comfortable, slow flow of heat from a
parafango pack, which retains its heat for a longer time
than other peloids (up to one and a half hours); burning is
not a problem even at this temperature.

Volcanic mud

Mud forms in places where the thermal waters from
volcanoes have chemically decomposed and become thermal
rocks and clay. This mud is a rich source of trace elements
and minerals that nourish the skin.

Moor mud

A famous therapeutic peat is Austrian Moor mud, formed
over 30 000 years ago in the Neydharting Moor by the
decomposition of vegetable matter. Its constituents include
over 1000 plants, 300 of which have medicinal, antibiotic
properties in addition to containing trace elements, phyto-
hormones, amino acids and vitamins. It is used for
abnormal skin conditions such as psoriasis and eczema,
sports injuries, joint and muscle problems, insomnia and
the relief of stress. Over 10 million **Moor peat baths** are
taken every year throughout the world.

Hungarian Wellness mud

This is a very fine therapeutic mud discovered in Kolop, 130 kilometres south east of Budapest and governed by the Hungarian Health Ministry (1956), whose regulations dictate that it is the only medical mud approved for use within all Hungarian medicinal spas. This sterile mud contains sulphate and iron. When heated it is excellent for the treatment of aches and pains caused by inflammatory and degenerative diseases of the joints.

White Thai mud

White coloured mud with a mineral composition of hydrated calcium sulphide is used in Thailand to cool down the skin, heal wounds, clear rashes and hydrate the skin.

Peat

Lowland peat is considered to be the best, especially from areas such as Austria. Body tissue has similar heat penetration, and although skin registers pain at a temperature of 42°C it can tolerate a hot peat pack at 45°C or a fango pack at 50°C. This is due to the heat transfer properties, which depend upon conductivity and storage ability. Research has shown that the optimum thickness of a pack is 5 cm. Female clients have reported an improvement in their skin after peat applications; these cosmetic effects are thought to be associated with tanning agents in the peat. Peat therapy is used in arthritis, soft tissue rheumatism, post joint surgery and for neck problems as a bath pack or ointment. Peat can be used over a wide range of temperatures from 4–50°C (see cold therapy, page 88). The Austrian company, Haslauer GmbH, produce a pack with a permeable membrane on one side which allows the peat to come into contact with the body.

Clay

Clay has been recognised through the centuries for its medicinal properties. Hippocrates used clay for healing wounds and poisonous lesions. Clays are composed of fine particles of specific rocks containing a large proportion of aluminium silicate. They are used to absorb and retain substances that are toxic to the body. Clay has a purgative effect when used internally and an exfoliating effect when used externally, leaving the skin very soft.

Medicinal earth

In the Rasul (treatment card 'Use and Application of the Rasul'), medicinal earths (muds) are used to draw out impurities from the skin. The medicinal properties from the earth are activated when massaged on to the skin, having a purgative and detoxifying effect, leaving the skin clean and soft.

Very fine-grained (white) earth is used on sensitive skin and on the face; fine-grained (red) earth is used on the chest, stomach and arms, and medium-grained (grey) muds are used on the legs, back and arms. Dark grey mud contains salt, which has bactericidal effects. The muds are natural in colour and are a result of the minerals present, i.e. red, and yellow muds contain ferric oxide.

Below is a list of medicinal earth (mud) used in the Rasul and recommended by the Austrian company, Haslauer GmbH.

- *Bolus alpha* – white; pure, very fine-grained, inorganic mud with good absorbing properties and very gentle desquamation.
- *Bolus beta* – yellow; pure, fine-grained inorganic mud with medium absorbing properties and gentle desquamation.
- *Bolus gamma* – red; pure, medium-grained, inorganic mud with low–medium absorbing properties and medium desquamation.
- *Bolus delta* – blue; pure, medium-grained, inorganic mud with high absorbing properties and medium desquamation.
- *Bolus epsilon* – grey; pure, medium-grained, inorganic mud with medium absorbing properties and high desquamation.
- *Bolus zeta* – dark grey; pure, large-grained, inorganic mud with stimulating properties, containing salt, high desquamation.
- *Bolus creta* – white; pure, very fine-grained, inorganic mud with very high absorbing properties.

Chalk (Rügen chalk)

Chalk has a finer grain than mud and an effective absorbing action that dries greasy skin. Iron oxides, chlorides and silicates from marble deposits are all found in chalk. The Romans recognised the healing properties of the lime of pulverised marble from Tinos and Carrara (NW Italy) and added it to their baths.

Fascinating Fact

One of the most popular treatments at the resort 'Les Sources de Caudalie Vinotherapy' in Bordeaux, France, is bathing in a barrel bath of natural hot spring water and the foam of the grape seed extracts, releasing free radicals from the body; another is 'honey and wine wrap'.

Silt

Silts found in inland lakes and coastal areas are rich in salts and are good for skin conditions such as psoriasis.

Loam

Loam is a rich soil consisting of a mixture of sand, clay and decaying organic material. It is used as an envelopment treatment in the Dry Float bed/Soft Pack system or as cold therapy packs. It has different thermophysical properties from peat and takes away heat from hot inflamed joints and other areas of inflammation and muscles.

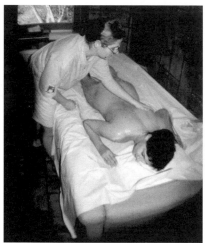

Haslauer GmbH, Germany

Vinotherapy

Vinotherapy

Vinotherapy is a treatment system that uses stabilised grape Polyphenols that are considered to combat the **free radicals** responsible for ageing. These treatments, using grape seed oil, grape extracts to the seed, stalk, wine yeast, skin and pulp combined with essential oils or clay, are thought to help decongest the tissues and boost circulation and to have a purifying, hydrating, relaxing or tonic effect on the body that strengthens the immune system.

They are used in body envelopment treatments, hydrotherapy baths, body scrubs, massage and facial treatments. To complete a treatment one is sometimes given a glass of wine – Chardonnay or Merlot for instance.

Alpine hay

This has a cleansing and gently stimulating effect that promotes blood circulation. It is good for rheumatic conditions and stimulates the immune system. It is gentler on the cardiovascular system than mud and fango treatments. The hay is either put directly and loosely all over the body (used in conjunction with Soft Pack system or Dry Float) or used as a compress over the liver and back treatment in the Kraxon bath.

Consultation process

The purpose of conducting a consultation is twofold:

1. Personal details.

2. Medical questionnaire.

The medical questionnaire is important because it will identify any medical problems which could be made worse (contra-indicated) by the treatments. It is also very important for medico-legal reasons to protect both the therapist and the client. The client's personal details are needed for business reasons and can also be utilised for further marketing and promotion.

The consultation allows the client to ask questions and breaks down the client/therapist barrier, thus creating a bond. Unfortunately, we are living in a 'blame culture', and there is a legal aspect to the completing of a consultation questionnaire. This will include an informed consent from the client/guest, who has been given an explanation of the treatment/product. This enables the client and the therapist to make a decision about the suitability of a particular treatment.

Overleaf is an example of a comprehensive chart of suggested consultation questions. Not *all* the questions are necessary for *every* treatment but there is a tick (in 'Observations') against the questions considered to be essential. Some spas address the issue of consultations by sending out a questionnaire in advance of the guest's arrival, thereby placing the onus on the guest to reveal any contra-indications to therapies, and where necessary, obtaining a doctor's approval for any proposed treatment. It is essential that the therapist reviews this questionnaire with the client prior to any treatment.

If the information and consent obtained is to be used for multiple visits, the medical questionnaire should be reviewed every 12 months. The document should include a clear request that any changes in the client's medical history, should be passed on to the spa reception and the relevant department.

The consultation process – rationale

Pregnancy

Many spas provide pregnancy programmes and water treatments in particular are excellent for relaxation for body, mind and spirit. However, a doctor should be consulted, as there is a risk that babies can miscarry – most frequently up to 14 weeks' gestation – therefore it is advisable not to give a treatment during this time.

Cardiovascular disease

In cases of mild to moderate heart failure water therapy can be beneficial as bathing removes water from the body via the kidneys. Water therapy is best avoided in severe congested heart failure.

CONSULTATION PROCESS	OBSERVATIONS
NAME	✓
ADDRESS	✓
	✓
Post code/zip	✓
Tel Home: Office:	✓
Fax:	✓
Mobile:	✓
Email:	✓
Website:	✓
Date of birth	✓
Occupation	✓
Doctor's name & tel:	✓
Your emergency contact number:	
Are you currently taking any medication?	✓
Are you taking any medicine which affects your circulation and ability to cope with heat – these include anti-coagulants, anti-histamines, stimulants, sedatives, vasoconstrictors and vasodilators?	✓
Have you had an operation or illness within the last 3 months?	✓
Are you currently undergoing another therapy?	✓
Do you wear contact lenses or spectacles?	✓
Known allergies:	✓
Iodine Seafood Garlic Pollen Bromine Chlorine	
Do you have a thyroid-related problem?	✓
Do you smoke? How many per day? Have you ever smoked?	✓
Any recent changes in bowel habit?	
What is your sleep pattern?	
Do you perspire easily?	
What sports do you participate in?	✓
Do you exercise regularly?	✓
Have you had a back injury? Do you suffer from back pains?	✓ ✓
Do you suffer from claustrophobia?	✓
Do you become tired easily?	✓
Are you nervous/anxious?	✓
Do you suffer from tension/stress/depression?	✓
Do you suffer from migraine?	
Do you know what is your trigger?	
Have you recently had a blood or cholesterol analysis?	

Do you have any of the following conditions – please specify and state medication:	
Diabetes	✓
Haemophilia	✓
IBS (irritable bowel syndrome)	✓
Colitis	✓
Acute diarrhoea – you should not use the spa within 48 hours of the symptoms subsiding	✓
Cancer (within 5 years)	✓
Endocrine disorder	✓
Uncontrolled epilepsy (recurrent fits despite medication)	✓
Cardiovascular disease (as severe heart failure, coronary disease, recent stroke or heart attack within 3 months), uncontrolled angina	✓
Thrombosis/DVT (deep vein thrombosis)	✓
Severe varicose veins	✓
Electrical implants: pacemaker/metal plates and pins	✓
Oedema – leg swelling	✓
High/low blood pressure	✓
Infected skin wounds and open sores	✓
Skin disease such as eczema or psoriasis	✓
Respiratory disease – asthma requiring regular inhaler use	✓
Unwell with a fever or infectious disease	✓
Recent sprains or muscle injury	✓
Have you any impairment of sensation e.g. from diabetes, stroke or injury?	✓
Are you aware of any circulatory problems such as cold hands or feet?	
Are you liable to nausea?	✓
Female questions:	
Are you pregnant or trying to get pregnant?	✓
Are you an IUD user?	✓
Are you menstruating?	✓
Nutrition:	
Eating patterns – regular intake/binges	
Do you eat between meals – if yes, what do you eat?	

Are you – vegan
      – vegetarian
      – wheat free
      – macro-biotic	

Do you have any food allergies?	
What is your daily fluid intake?	✓
What is your daily alcohol intake?	✓

How many glasses of water do you drink per day?	✓
Still or artificially carbonated?	✓
Do you have a lactose intolerance?	
Do you eat between meals?	
Do you eat foods with a high salt content – processed foods?	✓
Sodium intake – do you add salt to your food/cooking?	✓
What is your ideal weight?	
What is your weight?	
What is your height?	
Treatment objectives:	
What are your short-term goals?	
What are your long-term goals?	
What are your realistic expectations?	
Have you received a spa treatment before?	
Which treatment?	
Where?	
Evaluation record:	
Description of treatment	
Did the client enjoy the treatment?	
Are there any treatment procedure changes? Likes? Dislikes?	
Products used in treatment	
Recommended retail	
Therapist checklist. Have you:	
Made a physical assessment?	
Obtained medical approval if necessary?	
Explained the benefits of the treatment?	
Guided the client on critical safety points – i.e. emergency button?	
Gained the client's consent?	
Obtained the client's signature?	
After-care	
Treatment recommendations	
Product recommendations	
Which products would help to achieve their results/goals?	
The treatment plan to improve their results	
Rituals/home care	
Link therapies/treatments/combinations	
Any changes to be made	
Did they enjoy the treatment?	
Follow-up treatment/products/consultation	

Where there is coronary artery disease or recent coronary thrombosis (within 3–6 months), hot water treatments are contra-indicated. This is due to the increased vasodilatation, which increases blood flow in the skin and deprives the heart of blood. Hot water increases the viscosity of the blood, which could further precipitate clotting in those susceptible.

The heart action becomes less efficient in hot water above 38°C due to vasodilatation causing a temporary drop in blood pressure. This in turn, may cause low blood pressure, affecting the circulation to the brain, dizziness, either in the water or when standing up as gravity exaggerates the situation.

Deep vein thrombosis

Clients who have had deep vein thrombosis within 6 months are not recommended to have hot water treatments for fear of reoccurrence.

Cancer

Clients who have been treated for cancer within the previous five years must seek approval from their consultants prior to any treatment.

Because of the possibility of spreading cancer cells, no lymphatic drainage techniques should be performed on cancer patients. However, if the immune system is stimulated by hot or cold water treatments this is an advantage, as shown by the increased production of T4 cell lymphocytes. Gentle massage, as with an **aromatherapy** or affusion shower, can be beneficial to the well-being of the client – so long as the area around the tumour is avoided. This technique is already used with complete safety in some UK cancer units.

Skin diseases

Certain mineral waters and dilute brine are beneficial for eczema and psoriasis. The problem arises where the skin is cracked, as in severe eczema and psoriasis, because the brine acts as an irritant. Where the eczema is infected, psoriasis is present or where there is infection water treatments are to be avoided, as they may spread bacteria to other parts of the body or contaminate apparatus. Water temperature above 36°C in these conditions acts as an irritant.

Respiratory disease

Severe asthma that requires regular maximum dosage inhaler use can be exacerbated by sterilising agents such as bromine and chlorine in pools and baths.

Clients feels unwell with a fever

Hot baths raise fevers. However, research has shown that cold baths not only reduce a fever but stimulate the immune system, soothe aching muscles, increase the blood circulation to the brain and contribute to the overall improvement of the client.

High/low blood pressure

Blood pressure steadily rises with exercise; therefore strenuous exercise is contra-indicated where high blood pressure is present. In the case of high blood pressure, research work is conflicting, but some papers have suggested a rise in blood pressure in water-based treatments. Hot water increases the skin circulation, sometimes causing a drop in blood pressure and the onset of fainting and dizziness.

Infected skin wounds

Where there is infection in skin wounds, all water treatments should be avoided. See 'Skin Diseases', on the previous page.

Uncontrolled epilepsy

Epilepsy can be induced by hot water, flickering lights and reflections; therefore anyone who is subject to fits despite medication should not have warm or hot water-based treatments.

Diabetes

Diabetics whose condition is controlled by diet or tablets rarely have problems due to too little sugar (hypoglycaemia) or too much sugar in the blood (hyperglycaemia) or diabetic coma. However, those with insulin-controlled diabetes should observe the usual precautions, i.e. adequate food intake and a source of sugar handy in the event of a hypoglycaemic coma.

About 15 per cent of diabetics develop peripheral neuropathy where they lose sensation in their feet. This leads to injury as they lose the ability to feel changes in temperature and may burn themselves. The treatment should be terminated whenever any diabetic feels unwell.

Impaired sensation

Impaired sensation of the limbs or trunk can occur as a result of injury, stroke or diabetes (see previous page). Special care should be taken with these cases in spas.

Menstruation

Water treatments are contra-indicated in menstruation for hygiene purposes. Blood is a very good culture medium for bacteria.

Coil/IUD

Do not use the 'ventral ramp' (central stomach jet) of the hydrotherapy unit as it may cause the IUD to become displaced.

Complementary therapies

In orthodox medicine, hydrotherapy is employed to treat a wide range of disabilities, from rheumatic conditions and rehabilitation after stroke to sports injuries and post-operative conditions. In the field of complementary medicine, naturopathy and Kneipp treatments use water extensively. Therefore, it can be appreciated that spas bridge the gap between these two healing traditions.

The present authors believe that there is a place in spas for complementary therapies. Clients should be allowed access to such treatments, but the vital question is which ones? There is only room for a limited number in any spa and the spa manager is confronted by a whole range of possible complementary therapies.

The recent House of Lords Report in the UK – *Complementary and Alternative Medicine, a Report by the House of Lords Select Committee on Science and Technology* (November 2000) – raised the profile of complementary medicine whilst setting out a classification which stirred up considerable controversy. Basically, the committee chose between highly organised, scientifically proven, professional groups and those whose efficacy was in doubt scientifically and where training, codes of conduct and insurance cover were inadequate.

1. The report cited as core therapies: **chiropractic**, osteopathy, homeopathy, herbal medicine and acupuncture. These were deemed professionally organised alternative therapies, i.e. alternative to orthodox medicine, now that osteopathy and chiropractic have self-regulatory status by law and others are endeavouring to follow.

2. Included as 'complementary' therapies, i.e. to be used alongside orthodox medicine are Alexander Technique, aromatherapy, **Bach flower techniques**, bodywork therapies including massage, shiatsu, reflexology, healing, hypnotherapy, Maharishi Ayurvedic medicine, meditation, **nutritional medicine** and yoga.

3. In a third category were placed long-established therapies with a strong, specific, philosophical approach but which were 'indifferent to the scientific principles of conventional medicine' yet are said 'to give help and comfort to many'. These are: Ayurvedic medicine, Chinese herbal medicine, Eastern medicine, naturopathy and traditional Chinese medicine.

4. In the last part of this category (3B) were placed treatments 'lacking in any credible evidence base' and without adequate professional back up. These were: crystal therapy, dowsing, iridology, kinesiology and radionics. It is in these categories that there is controversy. Interestingly, the report did not refer to colour therapy at all.

The committee also set out the need for basic training standards, the need for continuing professional development and research, together with a knowledge of the limits of competence, where the practitioner should know when to refer cases onto another practitioner who may be able to help further.

The report only partially answers the question as which complementary treatments are most suitable for spas. One is left with the dilemma of whether to opt for core alternatives or complementary techniques. The authors consider that there should be a choice, possibly, from acupuncture, Alexander Technique, chiropractic and osteopathy, homeopathy and several types of massage chosen from classical Swedish, shiatsu, sports, Thai, Indian head or aromatherapy. Nutritional medicine and dietetics are increasingly important in this day and age of fast and highly processed foods. Dietetics should not be forgotten and should also be used in decisions about 'healthy eating' within spa catering.

Medical herbalism, counselling, naturopathy and clinical hypnotherapy should also be considered. For the larger spa with facilities to spare, the following therapies, though not essential, have an important place in an holistic-based spa: Ayurvedic medicine, Bach flower remedies, **cranio-sacral therapy**, **Reiki**, reflexology, traditional Chinese medicine and Chinese herbal medicine. Neuro-linguistic programming and colour therapy are also possibilities in a spa setting.

All spas should try to offer therapies from each category, except for the last (3B), where there is no scientific proof to back them up and little anecdotal evidence to support their claims. These 'fringe treatments' have no place in a modern spa which aims to present an honest and credible face to the public. Gimmickry costs credibility. It should not be forgotten that some treatments come and go with amazing frequency. In the healing arts this has always been the case, but some have stood the test of time, for example water therapies.

It is also important to have a balance between water-based treatments – the basis of a spa – and complementary therapies. The ratio of spa treatments, including hydrobaths, affusions, flotation, mud treatments, wraps, plunge pools, Watsu and Ai Chi, to complementary treatments should be 1:2 or 1:3. If a spa offers complementary therapies to clients, it is lacking in its duty not to advise which treatments would be suitable for an individual. To help tailor the client to the best regime for them requires a questionnaire and an advisor, not necessarily a particular practitioner, but a person who has been taught about the various treatments and has a working knowledge of them. It is very useful if these advisors have tried each of the treatments, so that they can speak from experience.

When employing a complementary practitioner it is important to ascertain that they have had adequate training and experience, are members of a recognised professional body with a recognised code of conduct and disciplinary procedure and possess adequate professional indemnity insurance. It is essential that every therapist is aware of his or her level of competence and knows when to refer to another practitioner or orthodox medical doctor. This is the case if the client fails to respond to treatment or the illness is life threatening, as with cancer, heart disease, and diabetes or severe allergies. Details of the plethora of professional bodies can be obtained from The Complementary Medicine Association, 142c Greenwich High Road, London SE10 8NN or www.the-cma.org.uk

Repeated customer surveys have pinpointed the most popular alternative treatments in the UK and Europe, but they are only a rough guide because of legal and cultural differences from country to country. For instance, massage

Fascinating Fact

Anthroposophical medicine was founded in the 1900s by an Austrian, Rudolf Steiner. It is practiced by qualified medical doctors and is particularly popular in Europe. It uses a holistic approach endeavouring to harmonise the spiritual and physical self. Techniques employed range from art, massage and hydrotherapy to eurythmy (movement therapy).

is very popular in Finland as is reflexology in Denmark, but Anthroposophical medicine, formulated by an Austrian, it is most frequently used in German-speaking countries.

Homeopathy has been tried most often in Belgium – by 56 per cent of the population. Osteopaths and chiropractors are commonly consulted, though more so in the UK, Sweden and the United States, where only 3 per cent of the population have used homeopathy and acupuncture. Another difference is that herbal medicine can only be practised by qualified doctors in most European countries, whereas in Great Britain therapists are non-medical. Thus, the complementary scene is not easy to evaluate accurately and usage varies widely across Europe. In the UK, the top five consistently popular complimentary therapies are: acupuncture, chiropractic, herbal medicine, homeopathy and osteopathy.

Acupuncture

Traditional acupuncture originated in China about 3500 years ago as a means of healing. It involves inserting fine needles into various energy points on channels called 'meridians', throughout the body. Twelve meridians run in pairs down the body, six on each side, corresponding to twelve major functions or 'organs' of the body, which are controlled by a vital force or energy called *qi* (pronounced 'chee').

Traditional Chinese medicine is concerned with the flow of *qi* and the balance of yin and yang, two opposite but complementary forces, essential to the well-being of the human body. It is the interaction of yin and yang that produces *qi*, the invisible 'life energy'. Acupuncture points situated along the meridians act as a means of controlling this flow of energy, which is blocked or unbalanced by disease.

The insertion of the needles is normally painless. The treatment is used mainly for pain relief in a number of conditions, especially in muscle and joint problems, migraine, addictions, asthma and hay fever, depression and anxiety.

There is some scientific evidence to support these claims and it has been noted that the needle insertions stimulate the release of the body's natural opiate production and other neurotransmitters (chemicals crossing brain connections and affecting brain function), such as serotonin, essential for mood control. This treatment is increasingly being used by orthodox medical practitioners and physiotherapists.

One of the variations of acupuncture is acupressure which has been succinctly described as 'acupuncture without needles'. This probably pre-dates acupuncture and is suitable for minor conditions, self-treatment and the indications for acupuncture, except for the treating of addictions. Another variant is auricular acupuncture. Each ear, according to Chinese medical theory, is said to possess over 120 acupoints relating to specific parts of the body. In auricular acupuncture, modern 'state of the art' therapists stimulate these sites by lasers and electrical currents or needles.

Osteopathy

An American, Doctor A. T. Still, devised osteopathy in 1872, in order to improve the healing capabilities of the body and the mobility of soft tissues and joints, especially those of the spinal column. The techniques employed are a mix of massage, gentle support of damaged tissues, releasing movements and manipulation, in contrast to the sudden, sharp manoeuvres of chiropractic. Like chiropractic, osteopathy is regulated by law in the UK and practitioners can only call themselves a chiropractor or osteopath if they are registered and properly trained. It is beneficial in conditions such as poor posture at work, through driving or due to pregnancy, repetitive strain injury and arthritis.

Some of its variations are *cranial osteopathy*, sometimes called *paediatric osteopathy* as it can help babies and young children with colic, irritability, insomnia or glue ear.

Chiropractic

Chiropractic evolved from osteopathy in 1898. It seeks to realign the bones of the spine that have been affected by what therapists believe are subluxations or small displacements. Treatment consists of sudden, sharp, short, manipulative movements called 'high velocity thrusts'. Though these are painless, they may produce a disconcerting 'click', which is nothing to worry about. Conditions treated include: poor posture, migraine, headaches, the pain from arthritis, sports injuries and accidents, trauma and stress.

Cranio-sacral therapy

Cranio-sacral therapy developed in the 1970s from cranial osteopathy. It involves gentle pressure on the upper (cranial junction) and lower spine or sacrum. This is said to be helpful in headaches, musculo-skeletal pain, dyslexia and learning difficulties.

Herbal medicine

Herbal medicine is sometimes referred to as **phytotherapy**. Herbs have been used as healing agents for 4500 years in India and China and later in Egypt, although English herbal books date from only the sixteenth century. Treatments are divided into Chinese, Western, Tibetan and Indian traditions.

Many conditions such as asthma, arthritis, eczema, migraine and menopausal symptoms are treatable by herbs but herbal remedies are not without risks as they may react adversely with conventional drugs, or be adulterated and contaminated with toxic materials; herbs should therefore be obtained from impeccable sources. Lastly, herbs contain a host of active ingredients and the strength and activity of these varies from batch to batch, so accurate dosing is difficult.

Western herbal practitioners have one main registering and regulating body – the National Institute of Medical Herbalists, which was set up in 1864. There is also a European Herbal Practitioners Association and a Register of Chinese Herbal practitioners.

Homeopathy

Dr Samuel Hahnmann set out his theory that 'like cures like' in a book entitled '*An Organon of Rational Medicine*', published in 1810. He believed that a medicine which causes the symptoms of an illness in a healthy person can cure that illness in an unhealthy one. Practitioners use naturally occurring substances diluted many times. Hence the title of a famous book trying to explain the homeopathic theory – *The Magic of the Minimum Dose*. Modern science cannot explain why, when the active substance is diluted so many times that there is hardly a molecule of it left, it still exerts a healing force. There are some 2000 remedies, which are used for 15 different constitutional types.

Practitioners use a holistic approach and take a detailed history in order to prescribe a medicine which is tailored to the individual and which must be taken in a certain way. Essential oils and certain drinks such as tea, coffee and alcohol interfere with this treatment.

Homeopathy is said to work best on children and adult chronic conditions such as eczema, rheumatoid arthritis, irritable bowel, mood disorders and recurrent infections of the upper respiratory tract and urinary system.

There are two types of practitioner – non-medical homeopaths and medically qualified ones.

Aromatherapy

Aromatherapy treatment uses aromatic essential oils distilled from the bark, leaves, petals, roots and stems of plants and trees that are known for their healing properties. Herbal oils made by infusion in castor or olive oil have been used since Biblical times.

In 1000 AD the Persian physician Avicenna developed a method of distillation and Crusaders brought the method back to Europe. By the Middle Ages essential oils were widely used for healing purposes and perfumes. In 1910 a French chemist noted how quickly his burnt hand healed when lavender oil was applied to it and a French doctor, Dr Jean Valnet, expanded this published work in the 1960s.

Essential oils are applied to the skin mixed with a carrier oil, as undiluted they cause severe irritation. According to modern research, the oils are absorbed through the skin pores in small quantities. Therapists use up to five oils in a mixture, tailored to the needs of the client, for a body massage. This has been found to induce deep relaxation, reduce anxiety, insomnia, headaches, asthma and to help solve gynaecological problems.

Reflexology

Foot massage has been used in China for over 5000 years. Reflexology was devised in 1915 by Dr W.H. Fitzgerald, who identified areas of the feet connected to ten energy zones throughout the body. Pressure on a reflex zone on the foot affected organs and tissues within that zone. The familiar 'organ map' of the feet and hands was physiotherapist Eunice Ingham's visualisation of Dr Fitzgerald's work. Reflexology is relaxing and helpful in insomnia, migraine, asthma, eczema, pain relief and high blood pressure.

Energy medicine

The idea that energy flows through the body by means of channels called 'meridians', stretches back to the origins of

Chinese and Vedic medicine. The 'subtle' energy therapies are often collected together under the term energy medicine. Health is thought to be related to the free flow of this energy and, where there are imbalances or energy blockages, ill health occurs. These energy-based therapies include:

- acupuncture
- colour therapy
- cranio-sacral therapy
- crystal healing
- homeopathy
- shiatsu
- sand therapy
- spiritual healing.

References

Camer, Richard H., 1999, 'Cyrotherapy', *Gale Encyclopedia of Alternative Medicine*, Gale Group, Gale Research.

Chiazzari, Suzy, 1998, *The Complete Book of Colour*, Element Books Limited, www.colourtherapyhealing.com

Franchimont, P. *et al*, 1983, 'CO2 Bath – Hydrotherapy – Mechanisms & Indications', *Pharmocology and Therapeutics*, 20, 79–93.

Hendy, Jenny, 2001, *Zen in your Garden, Creating Sacred Spaces*, Godsfield Press.

Hudson, Peter J., *The Moor, Natures Healing Miracle*, Mayfair Publishing, Eastbourne, East Sussex.

Kleinschmidt, J.G., 1988, 'Mud, mechanisms and effects of peat therapy', *Physikalische therapie in theorie und praxis* 10 October, 673–8.

Koelbl, Wolfgang and Ruth, *Transpersonal Soundtherapy*, Rogner Bad Blumau, Austria.

Ledingham, John and David Warrell (eds), 2000, *Concise Oxford Textbook of Medicine*, Oxford University Press, Oxford.

Swain, Liz, 2001, 'Sound therapy', *Gale Encyclopedia of Alternative Medicine*, Gale Group.

Useful addresses

Aura-Soma Products Ltd, South Road, Tetford, Horncastle, Lincolnshire LN9 6QB.

The Ayurvedic Institute, 11311 Menaul NE, Albuquerque, New Mexico 87112.

Bali Hyatt, PO Box 392, Sanur, Bali, Indonesia.

Brenner's Park Hotel and Spa, Schillerstrasse 4–6, D-76530 Baden-Baden.

Clavair, PO Box 2415, Maidenhead, Berkshire SL6 7WR.

Cymatics. www.telesound.co.uk

Danubius Hotel Gellért, Szent Gellért tér 1, H-1111 Budapest, Hungary.

Elemis Ltd, 57 The Broadway, Stanmore, Middlesex, HA7 4DU.

E'Spa, ESPA House, 21 East Street, Farnham, Surrey GU9 7SD.

Haslauer GmbH, Moosstrasse 131, A-5020 Salzburg, Austria.

HEAT Inc. PO Box 1177, Calistoga, CA 04515, USA – Reinhard Bergel, PhD.

Hyatt Hua Hin, Thailand

La Caudalie, France. www.caudalie.com

Le Meridien, PO Box 56560, CY-3308 Limassol, Cypress.

Nirvana Spa, Mole Road, Sindlesham, Wokingham, Berkshire RG41 5DJ.

Rogner Bad Blumau, Hotel and Spa, A-8283 Bad Blumau 100, Austria.

Rogner Héviz, Hotel and Spa Lotus Therme, H-8380 Heviz, Lotuszvirag u.Pf.80, Hungary.

Sound Healers Association, PO Box 2240, Boulder, Colorado, 80306 USA.

Thermarium, Schletterer GmbH, Bundesstrasse 154a, Jenbach, Austria.

The Spa, Hilton Hotel, Hua Hin, Thailand.

Tomatis Method. www.tomatis.com

Vinothérapie – Caudalie, Chemin de Smith Haut Lafitte, 33650 Bordeaux-Martillac, France.

Spa health and safety

5

Basic health and safety in a spa

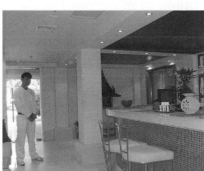

**The Spa reception at
The Hyatt, Hua Hin, Thailand**

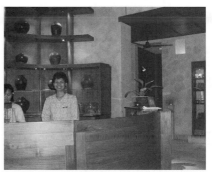

**The reception at The Spa,
The Four Seasons Hotel, Bali,
Indonesia**

Health and safety involves everyone working in a spa. The spa operator or manager is responsible in law, *in so far as it is reasonably possible*, for the health and safety of his employees and the general public using the facilities. In the UK, the relevant legislation is the Health and Safety at Work Act, 1974, and a number of other regulations, which will be discussed later.

Health and safety requires compliance with the regulations set down by a particular country. Different countries have different laws in this respect and each operator should check his or her country's regulations. Health and safety should begin at the planning stage of a spa.

Much of the regulations are common sense; some of them are blindingly obvious and boring. Nevertheless they are important. Just because they are obvious, they are easily forgotten and disregarded. Herein lies the danger. If these seemingly small points are overlooked someone may get hurt or even killed.

The main purpose of health and safety is to assess the risks of injury or illness occurring in the workplace and taking steps to minimise those risks. This in turn necessitates protecting both the employees in a spa and the general public who are using those facilities. It should be noted that even volunteer workers are covered by the legislation. To implement health and safety at work, thought must be given to a number of factors.

The spa manager should have authority to implement such measures as are necessary to ensure that every part of the spa premises is maintained at a high standard of cleanliness, hygiene and safety. Suggestions of ways to implement hygiene standards can be found at the end of this chapter in the form of examples of maintenance checks – Hourly, Morning and Evening Operational Cards. These include areas such as the filtration and disinfecting plant room, the storage and use of cleaning chemicals, the hazards of the pool, the various treatment suites, as well as the provision and presentation of food in the restaurant.

Risk assessment

Risk assessment is one of the most important parts of health and safety. It entails a careful evaluation of all the aspects of a spa that could cause harm to employees and to persons using the spa, in order to determine whether sufficient precautions are being taken to minimise the risks or whether more measures need to be put in place.

A risk is the chance, however great or small, of a person being adversely affected by a hazard. A hazard is anything which might cause harm. This may be anything from a slippery floor in a changing room or the decking by the poolside, to a chemical spillage in the plant room. The risk is the possibility of a fall on that floor or decking or the chances of a chemical catastrophe in the plant room. Most of the hazards are due to human error rather than mechanical fault or failure and the possibilities are almost limitless.

Removal of persons

Health and safety also involves appreciating how to remove from the building an injured person, or someone who has been taken ill, perhaps from an epileptic fit or heart attack. The removal must be done with the minimum of fuss and in such as way that will not exacerbate the injury or worsen the illness. In the case of fire or explosion an evacuation plan needs to be set out and practised in order to safely evacuate all the occupants of the spa.

Health and safety is practical

Many of the measures written in the regulations are qualified by the phrase, 'so far as is reasonably practicable'. This is important, as there is no point in setting out impracticable legislation. It is therefore up to the operator to ensure that

- the premises are made as safe as practically possible
- the staff have been adequately trained and instructed
- the staff are continuously and properly supervised.

How to assess a risk

In assessing a risk:

1. look for hazards everywhere

2. then think about those who may be harmed

3. balance the chances of harm being done

4. take appropriate action

5. record your findings

6. regularly review risk assessments.

7. where necessary make the appropriate changes.

Remember that in the UK it is mandatory to record the conclusions of a risk assessment where there are five or more staff employed. Check the rules in your country.

Spa managers should be taught to identify the hazards involved in running a spa and take steps to minimise the risks involved. In addition to training and record keeping, practical experience is fundamental to complying with the legal requirements. Good staff relationships are also essential to maintaining a safe spa with attentive staff who are motivated, competent and content. Staff should be taught basic hygiene rules, such as the importance of frequent hand washing, the use of fresh uniforms, regular washing of the poolside, bathing and treatment areas, and the proper storage, preparation and serving of food.

In the UK, health and safety inspectors and/or environmental health officers monitor all aspects of spa management.

UK regulations

The UK regulations that govern health and safety in the workplace, including spas, are listed overleaf.

Management of Health & Safety at Work Regulations (MHSWR) 1992

Spa operators have a duty of care to their employees and all users of their premises. Employers are required to:

- Carry out a risk assessment of the premises and treatments.
- Implement health and safety procedures to reduce the risks.
- Appoint competent persons to carry out the procedures.
- Set out emergency arrangements.
- Give information and thorough training to their workforce.
- Consult employees on these matters.

The risk assessment of the spa will need to include the physical hazards and those related to the local circumstances, such as different clients and groups, the equipment in use and the treatments given.

In order to formulate a policy for safe procedures, the following hazards and risks factors should be borne in mind:

- lack of, or inappropriate, supervision
- alcohol or food consumed before swimming or undergoing treatments
- clients with impaired sight or hearing
- pre-existing illnesses such as heart disease or uncontrolled epilepsy
- use of the facilities despite contra-indications
- disregard of warning notices
- age – remember that half those who drown are under 15 years of age
- poor or non-swimmers getting out of their depth
- slow or inappropriate response by staff to an emergency
- unauthorised use of a pool or treatment areas that are out of use
- misuse of equipment
- running along the poolside or diving into too shallow water, leading to concussion, head and spinal injury
- shallow diving should only be allowed where the minimum water depth is 1.5 metres and forward clearance is a minimum of 7.6 metres. Running

dives, backward dives, dives where the hands are not in front of the head, somersault and 'bombing' dives are all dangerous and should be prohibited.

The hazards encountered in spas have been evaluated. An American study found that of 158 deaths, only seven occurred in saunas; the remainder took place in spas, **hot tubs** and jacuzzis (Press, 1991). The risk factors were alcohol ingestion, heart disease, seizures and drug use (principally cocaine) with or without alcohol. These factors accounted for 71 (44 per cent) of fatalities; alcohol was the main cause in 38 per cent of cases; heart disease 31 per cent; seizures 17 per cent and drug-related deaths accounted for 14 per cent.

Surprisingly, in this study, 61 children under 12 years of age died in a spa environment; death was due to drowning from uncovered or improperly covered spas or through entrapment by suction.

A review of supervision in a spa forms part of a risk assessment

All pools need some form of supervision. The extent will depend on local circumstances, pool design and equipment and the nature of the groups using the facilities. Where individual baths and treatments are concerned, the therapist is the supervisor.

Lifeguards

The safe operation of a pool usually requires the use of lifeguards. Spa operators must ensure that lifeguards are adequately trained, effectively deployed, sufficient in number, alert and organised so that they are not unduly tired, stressed or bored when on duty.

A lifeguard should only be given that name if he or she has been adequately trained and is competent to carry out life-saving duties. Lifeguards can be employees, volunteers or attached to a group using the facilities or under a formal agreement made by the hirer of the spa. Operators must ensure that all lifeguards are competent, conform to the regulations, are properly supervised and understand their duties and areas of work

The supervision of programmed sessions involving the use of the facilities by groups or club must be considered. Where a teacher supervises school groups, lifeguard numbers may be reduced or dispensed with all together.

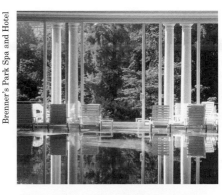

Brenner's Park Spa and Hotel

The pool at Brenner's Park Spa and Hotel, Baden-Baden, Germany

The safety of those with disabilities

This should be considered as part of the risk assessment and on a case-by-case basis. Operators should:

- consult with organisations and individuals who are in charge of disabled groups
- see that there are adequate facilities for getting into the water
- ensure that there are sufficient helpers in the water to look after the disabled – numbers will depend on the size of the group
- make sure that there are the appropriate warning signs, both visual and audible.

The supervision of children

As in any place used by the general public or by groups of persons, attention should be drawn to the problem of child abuse. Spa operators need to ensure that an effective system is in place to detect suspicious behaviour by adults towards children. Staff need to be aware of the problem, especially those supervising changing rooms, and be clear in their own minds what to do when inappropriate behaviour is noted. When such an occasion arises surveillance should be increased and the police and social services alerted. This applies both to in-house situations and where the facilities are hired out.

When recruiting new applicants for jobs, operators should seek information from previous employers regarding problems involving the supervision of children under 18 years of age. Information on past convictions, even if spent, should be obtained as restrictions regarding confidentiality are waived in the case of this age group, under the Rehabilitation of Offenders Act 1974.

Workplace (Health, Safety and Welfare) Regulations (WHSWR) 1992

This regulation deals with an extensive range of basic health, safety and welfare situations in the workplace, which apply to spas.

These regulations cover the following areas:

- temperature
- ventilation
- lighting

- cleanliness and waste materials
- room dimensions and space
- maintenance
- floors and traffic routes
- toilet, washing, staff changing and clothes storage facilities
- supply of fresh drinking water
- facilities for rest and eating meals.

Provision and Use of Work Equipment Regulations (PUWER) 1992

This regulation stipulates that:

1. Equipment supplied to the workplace is suitable, safe and correctly maintained for the employees' use.

2. Employees are competent in the safe operational use of the equipment.

3. Employees have sufficient knowledge of the equipment, including dealing with abnormal situations.

Construction (Design and Management) Regulations (CDM) 1994

These regulations apply to building projects, whether new, refurbishment and even demolition.

- Their aim is to improve health and safety, which is currently poor, through better management and design.
- These regulations describe documents, files and the duties of everyone, from clients and contractors to designers and the 'planning supervisor'.
- The regulations apply to any work lasting more than 30 days and using more than five people on site at any one time.
- They are a reminder that demolition and dismantling carry the greatest health and safety hazards.

Electricity at Work Regulations 1989

These regulations are a reminder that electricity is extremely dangerous in a pool or spa setting, where even a voltage as low as 50 volts can be lethal. This set of regulations cover the health and safety rules for the safe use of electricity at work and leisure in wet areas. They require that:

- All electrical installations and equipment are properly constructed and maintained and are correct for the purpose and environment in which they are used. This is important because of the humidity and wet conditions in a spa.

- The risks from the use of electricity – burns, shock, fire and injury from electrically activated equipment. These are all increased in the wet, humid and corrosive atmosphere of spas and pools.

- All electrical work – installation, extension and repairs – must be undertaken by specialist workers or supervised by those with specialist knowledge.

- Installation, extensions and repairs should also be carried out to a recognised standard, e.g. BS (British Standard) 7671.1992. This sets out the systems suitable for use in a spa or pool environment – which is complex – to avoid electric shock and which equipment should be used.

- Everyday electrical equipment, e.g. audio equipment at mains voltage, should not be used in wet areas unless specifically designed for use near water. Operators should make sure that third parties, e.g. trainers should not use unsuitable electrical apparatus in the spa. Specialist electrical equipment should be used in dry areas. Loudspeakers, electric clocks and other electrical apparatus must be placed out of reach of spa clients in any part of the wet facilities.

- The regulations state that the spa operator is responsible for seeing that all electrical installations are correctly carried out, effectively earthed and bonded where necessary.

- The efficiency of bonding and earthing should be visually inspected and tested every year.

- Switches should be fitted so that parts of an installation can be disconnected from the electrical supply.

- Socket outlets should not normally be located in wet areas. If they are in these environments they must conform to EN 60309-2:1998.

- The supply to wet locations should be protected to reduce electric shocks by the use of earth monitoring systems or RCDs (residual current devices) with a residual tripping current not more than 30 mA.

Specialist advice may be needed for the installation of RCDs.

- RCDs should:
  - be installed in damp-proof enclosures with sealed wiring
  - be protected against vibration and mechanical damage
  - be checked every day by firing the test button
  - be inspected visually with the equipment being used every week
  - be tested every three months by an electrician employing the appropriate test equipment.

- All electrical installations and equipment used in a potentially explosive atmosphere, for instance in the plant room where chemicals are stored and mixed or near an electrolyte sodium hypochlorite generator, should be suitable for use in such situations.

- Portable electrical apparatus should not normally be used in wet areas.

- To minimise the risks consider using

  - air-powered tools
  - battery-operated equipment
  - 50 volt tools from a safe extra low voltage (SELV) system
  - 110 volt tools from a reduced low voltage (RLV) system

- All electrical installations and equipment must be maintained in a safe condition, by periodic inspection and testing according to the manufacturer's instructions.

- Any unsafe apparatus must be disconnected and taken out of use.

- Formal visual inspections are important as they can detect up to 95 per cent damage or faults. These can be carried out by competent and trained staff, with adequate time to carry out proper surveys.

- Checks by the user should also be encouraged.

- Visual checks should include the removal of plug covers, confirming that the correct fuse is fitted, looking for evidence of overheating, loose wiring and corrosion.

- Electrical checks are required to find faults in insulation, earthing and contamination by dust or water. Visual inspection is unlikely to discover these types of problem.

- Keeping careful records of checks and maintenance.

Manual Handling Operations Regulations 1992

This set of regulations governs the movement of loads by hand. Spa operators need to assess the risks of manual handling. If risk is found to be present, these regulations apply:

- Avoid hazardous manual handling as much as possible.
- Assess the risk if this hazard cannot be by-passed.
- Reduce the risk of hazardous handling as much as possible.
- Review techniques that could reduce the risks.

Spa operators are responsible for these assessments and for reducing the risks to a minimum by altering the task, sharing the load with other workers or using a mechanical means of transportation. Employees are expected to:

- use equipment meant to increase safety
- adhere to safety systems for their work
- co-operate with management on all health and safety matters.

Control of Substances Hazardous to Health (COSHH) 1994

These regulations describe which substances are dangerous to heath, and how they should be used and stored. Most manufacturers issue clear guidelines and instructions.

The need for training

- As the disinfectants used in spas can be dangerous and even cause explosions, a knowledge of the chemicals involved and their interactions is essential.
- All employees should be made aware of the risks in using such substances and given training in the areas where they are used.
- Employees should also be familiar with the symbols and signs used to denote substances hazardous to health.
- Staff must be able to show that they are competent to maintain the safety of the plant.
- Training should also be given to spa and pool

managers so that they can supervise safe operations and deal with emergency situations.

- Details of training courses and attendees need to be recorded.
- Enough staff need to be trained so that it is never left to untrained staff to cope with an emergency situation.

Storage of chemicals

- Only trained staff should handle chemicals.
- There should be strictly no smoking in storage areas.
- There should be written procedures for dealing with these substances and a policy for:
  - labelling
  - display of safety notices
  - emergency situations
  - delivery and storage.

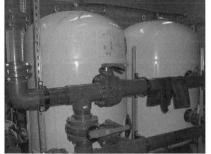

Storage procedures should incorporate the following measures:

- Different chemicals should be stored separately.
- Storage should be in a fire-resistant room (half an hour rated fire door), preferably with natural ventilation to the open air, and away from general public access.
- Where mechanical extraction or fans are used, these should be alarmed in case of failure.

Center Parcs, Aqua Sana

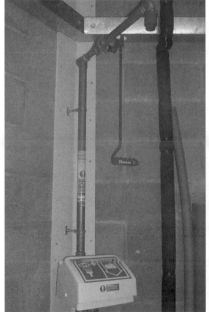
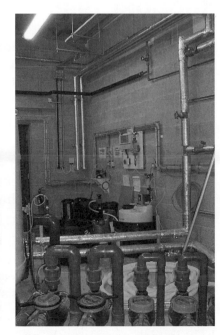
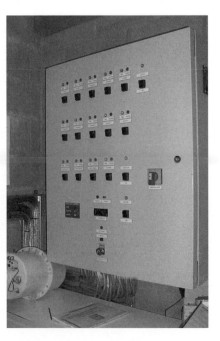

Storage of chemicals, Aqua Sana, Center Parcs Group, Longleat, UK

Emergencies may occur in the following situations:

- dangerous fumes may be emitted when chemicals are mixed together
- a fire can cause chemicals to overheat and emit fumes or explode
- explosions may occur when chemicals are mixed together
- where there is leakage from damaged containers
- explosion of pressurised containers.

A copy of the above regulations must be kept on the premises.

Employers must also make a formal assessment of the health risks, both to their employees and to the general public using the spa. One responsibility on employers is the requirement to use the 'least hazardous chemicals' that will produce the most satisfactory level of cleanliness.

It should be remembered that substances 'hazardous to health' also include the breakdown products of disinfectants and the interaction with contaminants brought in by bathers, for example sweat, mucus from the nose and lungs, urine, hair, cosmetics, skin lotions and sometimes faeces. Bacteria and viruses also form an important part of the hazards to health (see below).

Reporting of Injuries, Diseases and Dangerous Occurrences Regulations (RIDDOR) 1995

Under these regulations, within ten days of a work-related accident the operator of a spa is legally bound to report certain accidents to the Health and Safety Executive. These are:

- death of an employee, self-employed person or member of the public
- major injury sustained – fracture, dislocation, near-drowning, any person unconscious or hospital admission for longer than 24 hours
- member of the public taken to hospital
- 'dangerous occurrence', which may be a serious accident which does not lead to a reportable injury, e.g. lift failure, fire, electrical fault, explosion, or release of a hazardous substance.

It is advisable to record all accidents, however small, to help in risk assessments and provide information for RIDDOR at a later date.

Health and Safety (Safety Signs and Signals) Regulations 1996

This explains about signs and symbols. Any pool is safer if users are aware of potential hazards and they react responsibly to them. This can be done in the following ways:

- displaying notices at reception, changing rooms and poolside
- handing out a safety leaflet to clients as they arrive – but will they read it?
- giving leaflets to those in charge of groups
- providing oral reminders and warnings by staff, including lifeguards.

Examples of signs are:

- A responsible adult who can swim must accompany non-swimmers.
- No jumping or diving into the pool or running round the pool area for the safety and comfort of patrons and all pool users.
- For your comfort and safety do not swim within $1\frac{1}{2}$ hours after the consumption of food or alcohol.
- Remember it can be dangerous to swim alone.
- It is advisable to tie up long hair.
- In case of emergency – contact the nearest member of staff – activate the poolside alarm – use the poolside telephone to dial 999.

Decisions need to be made about where these notices are best placed and where they will be most easily seen – near the pool or in changing rooms and in the bedrooms of a destination spa.

Diving at Work Regulations 1997

Diving is not conducive to a relaxing spa environment and many spas ban diving altogether. However, UK Health & Safety Regulations allow shallow diving where the minimum depth of water is 1.5m with a forward clearance of at least 7.6m and a height of all surround above the water level not exceeding 0.38m. In pools where the depth is 1.5m, with unsupervised sessions the following dives are prohibited

- running dives
- backward dives
- dives where hands are not in front of the head

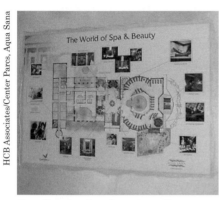

Spa Legend – showing the layout of the spa at Aqua Sana, Center Parcs, Longleat, UK.
www.centerparcs.com

- somersault dives
- indiscriminate dives, bombing or jumping.

It should be borne in mind that most spa pools are at a depth of 1.4m or less. The appropriate prohibition signs should be placed in pool areas.

Employers' Liability (Compulsory Insurance) 1969

Spa operators are responsible for the health and safety of their employees while they are at work. Employees may be injured or become ill whilst at work or as a result of present or past work. If an employee thinks the employer is liable, the employee may try to claim compensation. This act places a duty of care on employers to carry a minimum level of insurance against such claims.

This is different from Public Liability insurance which covers employers against claims made by members of the public. This type of insurance is voluntary, whereas Employer's Liability is compulsory.

Fire Precautions (Workplace) 1997

These regulations lay down minimum fire safety standards in the workplace. Spa operators must comply with them. If operators do not have control over parts of the workplace, there is a responsibility on the person or company who does. This is usually the owner or landlord.

Health and Safety (Enforcing Authority) Regulations 1998

These regulations divide enforcement responsibility for the Health & Safety at Work Acts (UK) between local authority and the Health & Safety Executive. These will obviously differ from country to country.

Personal Protective Equipment Regulations 1992

This legislation sets out the necessary personal equipment required when performing certain types of work and which must be provided by the operator. Suppliers of equipment and chemicals can help in this respect. The basic requirements are:

- dust masks
- face and eye protection
- aprons or chemical suits
- gauntlets
- boots.

In addition respirators may be needed where chemicals are mixed or where there is a likelihood of leakage of toxic gases, for example chlorine, bromine or ozone. Sufficient numbers of respirators need to be available in or near plant rooms. Respirators should be used as a last resort and replaced when their seals have been broken.

It should be noted that canister respirators can only cope with low concentrations of these gases. To deal with more serious leaks, the fire authorities should be consulted.

The Health and Safety (First Aid) Regulations (1981)

These regulations stipulate the minimum requirements for first aid in the workplace. These vary according to the number of employees and the nature of the facilities offered. However, there should be at least one employee with first aid skills and who possesses a current FAW (First Aid at Work) certificate – renewable every three years – on the premises.

The minimum requirements are a standard first aid box containing:

- a guidance card
- sterile dressings in various sizes
- adhesive dressings, individually wrapped, in various sizes
- eye pads
- safety pins
- triangular bandages.

The quantities will depend on the number of the workforce and throughput of the public. Other considerations are the type of treatments offered by the spa and the size and layout of the premises. The standard first aid box in a spa should be kept in a dust- and damp-proof container used only for this emergency purpose. It must be clearly labelled.

Because of the risk of falls and fractures, fracture boards and special stretchers, for example the scoop variety, should be available, as well as boards that float for recovery from swimming pools.

First aiders will have been trained in mouth-to-mouth resuscitation and CPR (cardio-pulmonary resuscitation), but it is advisable for as many as possible of the staff to be trained in this lifesaving technique through schemes such as Heart Start in the UK.

Further health and safety issues

Children in spas

This is a complicated problem, involving both health and safety considerations in addition to the practical aspects of spa management and the preservation of a calm ambience within the spa environment.

Drowning is the most common accident in spas involving children. Of 104 deaths reported to the Consumer Product Safety Commission in the USA, over half were children under 12 years old. In another study of 74 deaths of young children in Californian spas (Shinaberger *et al.*, 1990), the major factors involved were lack of supervision, access to the spa, neuromotor handicaps and entrapment.

Even with supervision, it is difficult to see small children because of their size, surface reflections and the reduced visibility due to steam.

- In whirlpools or a jacuzzi there is a greater risk for children of contracting infection from legionella, as the face of a small child is nearer the bubbling water surface and they are more liable to inhale the mists produced. These pools also operate at temperatures conducive for the growth of the legionella bacillus. For seated children to have their faces safely out of the water means that their average height should be at least 160 cms; this average is not attained until the end of the 10–15 year age group.

- Children tend to play about and dive under the water surface and thus may inhale or swallow infected water.

- Children have a less well-developed immune system than adults and are more liable to contract skin infections such as *Pseudomonas aerogina* which proliferate in these baths with a high bather load. These baths operate at temperatures at which certain bacterial growth is encouraged.

- Research studies (e.g. Shinaberger *et al.*, 1990) have shown that hot environments put a strain on the child's circulatory system in the following ways:

- Top (systolic) blood pressure remains static for all age groups, but declines in under 10-year-olds during the 4 minutes after leaving the sauna and then returns to its original level.
- Children under 10 suffered symptoms of dizziness (7 cases) and 2 out of 41 collapsed.
- There is a marked increase in heart rate.
- The cardiac reserve in young children is reduced.
- The ability to lose heat by transferring heat via the blood to the skin is reduced.
- The core body temperature of a child increases more quickly than in adults.
- Children have a higher metabolic rate than adults, which also acts to raise their temperature.
- The ability to lose heat by sweating is less well-developed in younger children. The young cannot control their body temperature as efficiently as adults can.

There are a number of environmental considerations:

- All children are active and tend to run and not walk. Getting them to sit still, for example in a whirlpool or steam room, is difficult as they soon get bored and move about.
- Their activity and boundless energy disturb the peaceful atmosphere of the spa environment. Adults come to spas to relax and a period of rest and quiet is required after treatments in order to obtain maximum benefit from them.
- Active children are more likely than adults to slip on wet surfaces surrounding pools.

There are also practical spa routine considerations:

- When a parent has booked a treatment, they should not take their children with them into treatment rooms, except in exceptional circumstances. The real answer to this is the provision of a crèche.
- The operator should set an age limit for children in a spa.
- All children should be accompanied by a responsible adult.

Food and drink in spas

Health and safety regulations also mention supervision where food and drink are consumed. Although they do not lay down hard and fast rules, supervision is required where food and drink are available in the same premises.

It is generally accepted that alcohol and complementary therapies do not mix, especially in the case of detoxification regimes, where the ingestion of alcohol actively works against the aims of the treatment. It is well known that alcohol and bathing are a dangerous combination and can lead to drowning and accidents.

Alcohol consumption should be banned or restricted until after treatments and prohibited between periods in water. Staff, especially those working in the restaurant areas and lifeguards should be on the look out for anyone under the increasing influence of alcohol. Another consideration in the alcohol debate is the risk of cuts and lacerations from broken glasses and bottles in a pool area.

Smoking in spas

A non-smoking policy is preferable in spas, because of health and fire hazards. Tobacco smoke pollutes the environment as well as people.

Hair care

In some European spas, male and female clients are not allowed to use the pools without tying up long hair or wearing a hair cap. This is not just for hygiene reasons, but it is also because long hair could become trapped in a water outlet.

These precautions and regulations are devised to minimise the risks of accidents and fatalities in spas. Adherence to them should ensure a safe spa, where clients can relax and enjoy their surroundings. The above regulations are those set out for the UK; other countries have variations on these rules and they must be checked in individual countries. We will now look at some example of legislation from other countries.

Overseas regulations

Asia

In Hong Kong, public swimming pool regulations are made under section 42 of the Public Health and Municipal Services Ordinance, Chapter 132, Section 149(1) of that ordinance.

Chapter 132BR Public Swimming Pools Regulation, Section 8.

Gazette Number LN320 of 1999, Version date 01/01/2000.

Personal Hygiene.

'No person shall enter a swimming pool without first having passed through a shower and foot bath.'

These regulations also have an Empowering Section.

Canada

In the state of Alberta, a licence is required to operate a swimming pool.

AR 247/85 Swimming Pool (consolidated up to 251/2001)

Alberta Regulation 247/85, Public Health Act, Swimming Pool Regulation.

They define 'public swimming pool' for public use and 'semi-public pool' as being provided by a hotel, club, educational institution, apartment building or mobile home park. This is defined further as pools operated in conjunction with recreational camps, care institutions for the aged or infirm.

An application for a licence must include the following information:

- the source of the water supply
- the method of waste water disposal
- the diving, swimming and deck areas
- the pool volume
- the maximum design bathing load
- the design circulation rate
- the chlorinator capacity
- the filter area and type.

A local board may apply terms and conditions to the licence and the licence remains the property of the local issuing board.

A notice board has to be conspicuously placed listing the rules and regulations, such as:

- Persons are required to take a cleansing shower prior to using the pool.
- It is prohibited to spit in, spout water in, blow the nose in, urinate or pollute the water.

Other regulations cover the changing rooms, floors, furniture, materials used, food and beverages and more.

France

There are no safety regulations for swimming pools built in private homes or for hotel and resorts, however this is changing. The Security and Quality Department for Consumers of the French Ministry of Economics, Finance & Industry is currently producing legislation for swimming pools.

Ministère de l'Economie des Finances et de l'Industrie
Service de la Consommation, de la Qualité et de la Sécurité
59, boulevard Vincent Auriol
75703 Paris Cedex 13, France
Tel: +33 1 44 97 23 81

First aid in spas

The authors recommend that all spa personnel be trained in first aid (see Health & Safety (First Aid) Regulations (1981)). Summon a first aider or medical aid as soon as this is necessary. Below are some brief notes for the untrained first aider.

Minor cuts

Cover with a sterile dressing and apply pressure to stop bleeding.

Severe cuts

Where bleeding is profuse, apply pressure with a clean towel or sterile dressing. If blood seeps through dressing apply another on top. Do not remove first dressing as this disturbs natural clot formation and encourages further bleeding. Wear surgical gloves wherever possible to avoid contact with blood.

Bruises

Bleeding into the skin and underlying tissues causes bruises. Treatment aims to minimise this by elevating the affected part and applying a cold compress or ice pack for five minutes at a time.

Sprains

Soft tissue injuries:

- A *sprain* is an injury to a ligament, at or near a joint.

- A *strain* is the over-stretching of a muscle, which commonly occurs in athletes.
- A *rupture* is a complete tear of muscle tissue or ligament.

Treatment is summarised in the word RICE:

R **rest** the injured part
I apply **ice** or a cold compress
C **compress** and apply gentle pressure by padding and bandaging to the injured area
E **elevate** the injured area, to reduce blood flow and bleeding into the surrounding tissues.

If the injury is severe there may be a broken bone (fracture) at the site of the injury.

Fractures

If in doubt about the severity of an injury, treat as if it were a fracture, by supporting the injured part and immobilise by securing the injured area to a undamaged part of the body — for example upper limbs to the chest wall with a sling or bandage, and the lower limb bandaged to the other leg.

Dislocation

This occurs when a joint bone is forced partly or completely out of its socket. This commonly affects shoulder, thumb or jaw joints and may be associated with fracture or ligament damage. Dislocation of the spine is very serious as any movement may result in paralysis. Medical aid should be urgently sought.

Dizziness

This is usually due to a lack of blood to the brain. Sit the person down and help them to put their head between their knees to encourage blood to return to the brain. There are other more serious causes for dizziness, so it needs to be ascertained if the person is subject to these attacks and whether medication is being prescribed.

Fainting

This is also due to a lack of blood to the brain. Lie the client down on the floor and raise both legs to encourage the blood to return to the head. Consciousness should return within a minute or two. If this does not happen summon medical aid.

Nosebleed

First lean the head forward, preferably over a washbasin or receptacle and persuade the sufferer to breathe through their mouth whilst pinching the soft tip of the nose in order to stop the blood flow – this may take 20 minutes or longer.

Falls

Ascertain the severity of the damage. If the person complains of severe back or neck pain or cannot move without pain, cover them with a blanket. Do not attempt to move them. Summon medical aid.

Asthma

Remove the wheezing and distressed client from the area into fresh air. Allow the client to use their inhaler. Place them into a comfortable position where breathing is easier – sitting up and slightly forward, with arms leaning on something firm, such as the back of a chair. In mild cases if there is no improvement in 15 minutes, repeat inhaler use.

Obtain medical aid if attack is severe or getting worse and there is no improvement 5 minutes after inhaler.

Epilepsy

Remove anything in the vicinity which may harm the client during the convulsions. Ensure that the person is not choking on their tongue and that their air passages are clear. Do not try to restrain, as this will only exacerbate the attack and the spasms. Wipe froth from the mouth. After the spasms have ceased, cover them with a blanket, place in the 'recovery position' and allow them to rest or sleep. Do not leave them alone until fully recovered and watch out for a period of automatism (lack of conscious control).

Unconsciousness

Place anyone who has lost consciousness on their side in the 'recovery position' as shown in first aid manuals. Request medical help immediately. If breathing has ceased, give mouth-to-mouth resuscitation. If the heart has also stopped, give cardio-pulmonary resuscitation (CPR).

Drowning

Remove the person from the water, endeavouring to keep their head lower than the rest of the body to avoid further inhalation of water through vomiting. Lay casualty on their back on a firm surface; use swimming pool stretcher if available. If unconscious check that mouth is clear of any obstruction. Give rescue breaths if not breathing and continue to do mouth-to-mouth resuscitation and if no signs of a heart beat, give chest compressions. Summon medical aid. Keep casualty warm by covering with a blanket.

Burns

Hold the affected area under cold running water or immerse in cold water until the pain is relieved. Where there is blistering or broken skin involving a significant area of the body, cover with a sterile non-stick dressing and seek medical aid.

Electric shock

Switch off electric current before touching or removing casualty from area. Remember that electricity can 'jump' from the casualty to the rescuer if the current is not switched off. Treat any burns. Cover with blanket. Request urgent medical aid.

Foreign bodies in the eye

Use the corner of a handkerchief or, preferably, a twist of sterile cotton wool, or the corner of a sterile dressing, and try to draw foreign body from surface of the eyeball to the corner of the eye. Flush eye with sterile water.

Chemical spillage into the eye

Immediately flush eyes with sterile water from wash bottle or use an eye bath. Seek medical aid.

Waterborne infections

Showers taken prior to swimming or any water therapy effectively reduce the frequency and severity of waterborne infections. Foot baths are barriers to the outside world, preventing the entrance of dirt into a spa, but they are of very limited use in combating infections, foot sprays or showers have been proved to be a more efficient way of removing body surface contaminants, for example body lotions, creams, oils and dead skin.

The following waterborne infections are listed in alphabetical order and not in order of frequency of occurrence.

Acanthamoeba

These amoebas, sometimes isolated from bathing waters, have rarely caused infections linked to spa pools. This organism can contaminate contact lenses and cause ulcers on the cornea.

Adenoviruses

These viruses in poorly disinfected pools can cause pharyngoconjunctival fever characterised by a sore throat, red eyes and fever.

Cryptosporidium parvum

These protozoa, chemically and physically robust and resistant to chlorine but not to filtration, are the commonest cause of diarrhoea in pools. Disinfectants reduce oocysts' viability but do not remove them. Ozone and UV can be effective.

Dermatophyte fungi

Athlete's foot (*Tinea pedis*) can be caught from floor surfaces contaminated by fungus-laden skin fragments. It causes itching and scaling between the toes, which often looks like soggy skin so the diagnosis is sometimes difficult. Frequent floor cleaning reduces the incidence.

People with severe infections should be excluded from bathing. However, it is not practicable to exclude everyone with a mild infection. Footbaths are not effective in stopping the spread of infection, however, it is thought that foot showers with a disinfectant are effective. Surprisingly, children do not usually get athlete's foot. The fungus is not killed by chlorine.

Escherichia coli (commonly known as E-coli)

These bacteria are spread mainly through food and from person to person. One outbreak in the UK resulted from a poorly disinfected paddling pool. It is killed by adequate chlorination.

Giardia lamblia

This protozoa has similar characteristics to *Cryptosporidium parvum*.

Hepatitis A virus

The Hepatitis A virus causes infectious inflammation of the liver and is spread through contaminated food and water, but is killed by chlorine.

Legionella pneumophila

A respiratory infection spread by bacteria in aerosols or sprays which can be a problem in spas. It is also present in biofilms (slime) which builds up in the pipe work of spa baths. Fortunately, this bacillus is killed by chlorine.

What is legionnaires disease?

This is a form of pneumonia which kills about 12 per cent of those infected. It is caused by the legionella bacteria, which can also cause flu-like symptoms, fever, chills, headache and muscular pain. Legionnaires disease usually develops 3–6 days after exposure. About 30 per cent of those infected will develop diarrhoea or vomiting and 50 per cent become confused or delirious.

How does legionnaires disease develop?

It is caught by breathing an invisible aerosol containing legionella bacteria. Aerosols can be formed from tiny droplets generated from water containing the bacteria, for example bubbles rising through water in a spa pool, misting systems, water features, fountains and showers. Water drawn from a stagnant source and, when these have not been used for a long time, running a tap or flushing a toilet can also spread the bacteria.

The bacteria can live and multiply in water at temperatures of 20–45°C. They can be found in the natural environment such as rivers, lakes and moist soil.

This disease *cannot* be caught from another person.

Legal responsibilities

The Health & Safety at Work Act 1974 and the Control of Substances Hazardous to Health Regulations 1999 relate to preventing the risk of exposure to legionella bacteria, the cause of legionnaires disease. If you use water in your equipment or display you must have a written risk assessment for legionella control.

Key risk factors encouraging legionella:

- warm water between 20°C and 45°C
- spray/mist/bubble formation
- recirculating water – spa pools
- water left untreated at 20°C and 45°C
- biofilm (slime) and dirt on pipes, tubing and tank/container surfaces
- stagnant water encouraging the growth of a biofilm
- washers and seals.

The following measures will reduce these risks:

- keep equipment clean and free from scale
- use a chlorine-based disinfectant
- store equipment dry
- clean and disinfect pipes and filters at regular intervals
- spa baths (whirlpools): check filters daily; check water treatments at least three times daily; clean and disinfect
- use a swimming pool test kit
- keep daily records of all water treatment readings, such as temperature and chlorine concentrations.

Leptospira

Bacteria from the urine of infected rats and other animals in rivers and lakes, which cause Weil's disease. This disease is characterised by jaundice, meningitis and kidney failure. Adequate chlorination kills the bacterium.

Mycobacterium marium

This bacterium, occasionally found in pools and killed by adequate chlorination, causes a very rare skin condition – swimming pool granuloma, which is a warty or pustular lesion.

Naegleria fowleri

This is an amoeba, which can cause meningitis in swimmers who have dived or swum underwater or inhaled infected spray. It is found in thermal spring water worldwide, but there is no problem with mains water because of its lower temperature and chlorination. It can encyst and become resistant to disinfectants. Prevention by using an uncontaminated source of thermal water is the best line of treatment.

Papilloma virus

Plantar warts (verrucas) are caused by contact with floors and surfaces contaminated by the virus, which is not killed by chlorine.

Pseudomonas aeruginosa

A bacterium predominantly affecting spa pools and occasionally found in swimming pools. Though killed by chlorine, heavy contamination in poorly run pools can cause inflammation of skin follicles (folliculitis) and ear infections (swimmer's ear).

Shigella

This bacterium, rendered harmless by chlorine, causes dysentery in poorly run pools.

Trichobilharzia schistosoma

A flatworm parasite (shistosomes) causing swimmers' itch – found in lakes and coastal beaches containing snails and birds. This parasite penetrates the skin whereupon it dies, but in one-third of contacts, an allergic reaction occurs. This reaction lasts for about one week.

Waterborne illnesses in spas and swimming pools

Skin rashes

Skin rashes are usually due to the degreasing action of water and subsequent wetting of the skin. Degreasing is the action of almost every disinfectant. Disturbance of the skin barrier occurs with prolonged immersion in warm and hot water and allows chemical irritation and infection to occur. The differences between a chemical cause and an infection are:

- *Chemical irritation* – invariably due to bromine-based disinfectants, e.g. bromochlorodimethylhydantoin (BCDMH). Rarely occurs with chlorine and is then mild. Occurs immediately or within 12 hours; itching is severe.

- *Infection* – bacterial infection may cause inflammation of hair follicles (folliculitis). More likely in spa pools or whirlpools. The bacterium is *Pseudomonas aeruginosa*, occurring in water above 32°C and when exposure is 1–2 hours. Symptoms develop after 24 hours; itching is mild to moderate. Viral infection causes plantar warts. Children are usually affected, as adults have acquired immunity.

Nose and sinus (cavities in the bones of the face, above and below the eyes) problems may be due to chemical irritation or pressure changes due to diving and underwater activity or osmotic pressure effects. Infections due to swimming or water treatments are unusual.

Disinfection

The maintenance of disinfectant levels may be influenced by different elements:

- elevated temperatures
- amount of sunlight present
- high turbulence caused by the hydrotherapy jets
- aeration, high organic loading due to heavy use.

The following disinfectants or combinations may be used in spa water:

- bromochlorodimethylhydantoin
- chloroisocyanurates
- sodium hypochlorite
- calcium hypochlorite
- ozone in conjunction with a residual disinfectant, e.g. sodium hypochlorite or calcium hypochlorite.

Cautions

High levels of dosing may cause irritation to the mucous membrane of the eyes and throat. This can be avoided by keeping the combined chlorine concentration below 1 mg/L. No disinfectant will work efficiently if there is an accumulation of organic matter in the strainers, filters and pipe work.

Bromochlorodimethylhydantoin

This is added from a dosing unit – 100 mg/L; excessive concentrations are associated with skin rashes. The undiluted compound can cause severe burns on contact with skin and eyes. It should not be mixed with other chemicals and it reacts with oxidisable material such as solvents, wood, paper and oil.

Chloroisocyanurates

This is available as slowly dissolving tablets (trichloroisocyanuric acid – automatic dosing unit) or rapidly soluble white granules (sodium dichloroisocyanurate – dosed directly into spa pool).

When wet, chlorinated isocyanates liberate toxic chlorine gas and are liable to explode. Concentrations should be maintained below 200 mg/L. Cyanuric acid concentrations above 200 mg/L can encourage algal growth.

Sodium hypochlorite

This is supplied as a solution with a concentration of 12–15 per cent available chlorine and requires dilution. The active disinfectant is hypochlorous acid. When mixed with acids, it produces toxic chlorine gas.

Calcium hypochlorite

This is supplied as a powder or in granules and must be dissolved prior to use. The active disinfectant is hypochlorous acid and more frequent backwashing of filters are needed due to deposition of calcium salts. When mixed with acids, it produces toxic chlorine gas.

Ozone

Ozone should only be used with a residual disinfectant. The type of ozonisation depends upon the spa installation. Free chlorine residuals will still need to be maintained above 1mg/L – ideally between 2–3 mg/L.

Ultraviolet light

Ultraviolet light is known to have a bactericidal effect, however, additional disinfection is required by an oxidising biocide, for example chlorine. The UV lamp needs to be checked daily to ensure it is operating.

Filtration

The filtration system design is linked to circulation pumps, heaters, pipe work and valves, etc. Filters remove particles of matter, either suspended or in colloidal form, from pool water. They should run continuously to combat the pollution derived from bathers, however, they may have a reduced flow rate at night.

With inadequate or ineffective filters, the build up of suspended solids increases turbidity. This reduces the clarity of the water, which is critical. With properly filtered water it should be easy to see the bottom of the pool. If the bottom cannot be seen, there is a high chance of discomfort to bathers. Reduced clarity makes it difficult to see anyone in distress, for example a small body.

Cheap filters should be avoided, as they are unable to cope with the large bather loads. Experience in spas suggests that sand filters are the most efficient. Coagulants, or flocculants as they are sometimes called, aid the removal of suspended or colloidal material. They work by bringing the pollutants out of solution or suspension as solids. This is coagulation. When the solids clump together producing a floc which is easily trapped inside a filter, the process is called is flocculation.

The most important use of coagulants is in trapping bacteria, the infective cysts of cryptosporidium and giardia which are resistant to disinfectant, humic acid and phosphates, all of which would otherwise pass through the filter.

Where pH values are above the recommended range, coagulants are less effective and a minimum alkalinity of about 75mg per litre of $CaCO_3$ (calcium carbonate) is required for effective flocculation.

Ozone breaks down colloids and is most effective when applied to water treated with a coagulant and filtered. Aluminium-based coagulants are most commonly used.

Linings, if needed, can be a problem if the materials and their application are not properly addressed.

Water treatment

These are some of the considerations when handling water in a spa:

- Design considerations.
- Water source/guidelines on water quality.
- Pool type/pool temperature.
- Filtration/disinfection/oxidising agents/pH adjustment.
- Water balance/fresh water dilution.
- Water testing and recording.
- Effects on air quality.
- Plant size and operation.
- Plant monitoring and control/personnel and training.
- Energy and operational costs.
- Microbiology.
- Introduce routine testing and recording.
- Pool is operating within the limits of pool design.
- Bathing load, filtration rate, dilution.

Water testing

The following are invaluable aids to water testing in a spa:

- Material safety data sheets.
- Identification of substance and manufacturer.
- Composition/ingredient information.
- Hazards identification.
- First aid measures.
- Fire-fighting measures.
- Accidental release measures.
- Handling and storage.
- Exposure controls.
- Chemical properties.
- Stability/reactivity.
- Toxicological information.
- Ecological information.
- Disposal information.
- Transport information.
- Regulatory information.
- Other information.

The Hourly Operations Instruction Card

By: Jane Crebbin-Bailey HCB Associates

Every hour the spa attendant should check the following:

Greek herbal hath

- The steam is generating in the Greek herbal bath
- The floor inside and in the surrounding area is clean and any surface water is removed
- Remove any discarded towels and paper cups
- Clean the benches with water using the Kneipp hose and a suitable disinfectant, to ensure hygiene standards are maintained

The Turkish hamman

- The steam is generating in the steam room
- The floor inside and in the surrounding area is clean and any surface water is removed
- Remove any discarded towels and paper cups

Experience showers

- The shower heads are operating efficiently and are not clogged
- The floor inside and in the surrounding area is clean and any surface water is removed
- Remove any discarded towels
- Clean the showers with a suitable disinfectant, to ensure hygiene standards are maintained

The reflexology footbaths

- The floor inside and in the surrounding area is clean and any surface water is removed
- Remove any discarded towels and paper cups
- Clean the basins and benches with a suitable disinfectant, to ensure hygiene standards are maintained

The laconium

- The floor inside and in the surrounding area is clean and any surface water is removed
- Remove any discarded towels and paper cups
- Clean the benches with water using the Kneipp hose and a suitable disinfectant, to ensure hygiene standards are maintained

Tyrolean sauna

- Check the Tyrolean sauna temperature and remove any discarded towels
- Refill the bucket with clean water and ladle 5 scoops of water on to the coals

The ice room

- The floor inside and in the surrounding area is clean and any surface water is removed
- Remove any discarded towels and paper cups
- Break up the ice in the centre bowl
- Clean edge of bowl and ledges

The meditation room

- The floor inside and in the surrounding area is clean
- Remove any discarded towels and paper cups
- Clean the ergonomic couches with a suitable disinfectant, to ensure hygiene standards are maintained
- Ensure that the music is not too loud
- Ensure that the lighting is dimmed
- Ensure that the aromatic burners have water and essential oil in the top of the burner to stop the bowl from cracking

Japanese salt bath

- The floor inside and in the surrounding area is clean and any surface water is removed
- Remove any discarded towels and paper cups
- Clean the benches and centrepiece with water using the Kneipp hose and a limescale remover, to remove salt stains and to ensure hygiene standards are maintained
- Wash the stones in the centre bowl with a suitable proprietary cleaning agent to remove any algae build-up

Morning Operations Instruction Sheet
By: Jane Crebbin-Bailey HCB Associates

Cleopatra slipper bath

Morning
1. Check the pool and jets are clean
2. Remove any towels, robes or paper cups
3. Ensure that the surrounding area is clean and dry
4. Prepare the aromatic burner and candles

Standard cleaning programme
The Cleopatra slipper pool should be cleaned with a suitable non-abrasive proprietary cleaner

NB *Ensure the aromatic burner and candles are lit*

Aqua meditation room

Morning
1. Check the heated benches are on – switch located in plant room
2. Press the **green** button and the light will illuminate. This will turn on the heating
3. Remove any towels, robes or paper cups
4. Ensure the mirrored glass in fountain is clean
5. Check that the fountain – top and base – has been replenished with clean water
6. Check that the leather-style heated benches have been cleaned with a suitable proprietary cleaner to ensure hygiene standards are maintained
7. Ensure the music is not too loud
8. Check the lights in the fountain are operating
9. Check the water inlets in the ceiling are operating correctly
10. Check level of essence in bottle (lemon) – located in plant room
    NB *Unscrew and replace with new bottle of essence*
11. Ensure the floor is clean and any surface water is removed

Standard cleaning programme
The aqua meditation room should be cleaned with sponges

Indian blossom steam room

Morning
1. Check the heated benches are on – switch located in plant room
2. Press the **green** button and the light will illuminate. This will turn on the heating
3. Remove any towels, robes or paper cups
4. Enter the Indian blossom steam room and spray the walls, benches and floor with the Kneipp hose
5. Check the level of essence in bottle (ylang-ylang) – located in plant room
   NB *Unscrew and replace with new bottle of essence*
6. Check the fibre optic lighting is operating

Standard cleaning programme
The Indian Blossom Steam Room should be cleaned with a combination of bristle brushes on the mosaic surfaces and sponges for the tiles

NB *Deposits of calcium and scale may form on surfaces. A proprietary cleaning agent should be used each evening to avoid unsightly staining*

Morning Operations Instruction Sheet
By: Jane Crebbin-Bailey HCB Associates

Relaxation/meditation room

Morning
1. Check the ceramic heated couches are on – switch located in plant room on the main control panel
2. Remove any discarded towels and paper cups from the meditation room
3. Close the door of the meditation room to allow the room to reach its operating temperature
4. Ensure that the lighting is dimmed
5. Ensure that the aromatic burners have water and essential oil in the top of the burner to stop the bowl from cracking
6. Ensure that the music is not too loud
7. The floor inside and in the surrounding area is clean
8. Check that the ergonomic ceramic heated couches have been cleaned with a suitable disinfectant, to ensure hygiene standards are maintained
   (When switching on in the morning, it will take approximately 2 hours to reach this operating temperature)

Reflexology footbaths

Morning
1. Check the reflexology footbaths are on and operating correctly
2. Remove any discarded towels and paper cups
3. Check the floor in the surrounding area is clean and any surface water is removed

Ice fountain

Morning
1. Check the ice fountain is producing ice
2. Remove any discarded towels and paper cups
3. Check the floor in the surrounding area is clean and any surface water is removed
4. Check the temperature. This should be 15°C
5. Break up the ice in the centre bowl
6. Clean edge of bowl and ledges of centre bowl
7. Check that the ice release sensors are not blocked

Morning Operations Instruction Sheet
By: Jane Crebbin-Bailey HCB Associates

Serail

Morning

1. Turn on Serail cleaning light – located in plant room
2. Turn on the Serail, one hour prior to first guest – switch located in the plant room
Press the **green** button and the light will illuminate
NB *This will allow the walls, floor and benches to heat to the correct operating temperature*
3. Turn on the steam generator
4. Check levels of essence bottle and change if empty
NB *Unscrew and replace with new bottle of essence*
5. Enter the Serail and check the fibre optic lighting is on, that the Serail is clean and that all towels have been removed
6. Press on **ALL** the 'head shower' buttons in each alcove to ensure that warm water is drawn from the boiler and ready for the first guest. Then press on **ALL** the side jets
NB *If one of the buttons on the showers fails to operate, it may be due to damaged or worn bellows. Please advise the maintenance engineer as soon as possible*
7. Close the door to allow the room to reach operating temperature
8. Check the temperature on the main control panel, this should be 35–45°C
9. Once the guests have left the Serail, remove all the mud bowls and towels and close the door
10. Turn on the cleaning button located outside the Serail
NB *This activates the automatic cleaning cycle that sprays water around the room. This process takes 2 minutes. When the cycle is completed re-enter the Serail and clean the benches in the alcoves, central basin and floor with a disinfectant. Use the Kneipp hose for extra water. Keep the door closed during cleaning to maintain the temperature of the Serail for subsequent guests*
11. Exit the Serail and turn off the cleaning light

Greek herbal bath

Morning

1. Check the Greek herbal bath is on – switch located in the plant room on the main control panel
Press the **green** button and the light will illuminate. This will turn on the heating.
2. Turn on the fibre optic lights
3. Turn on the Greek herbal bath one hour prior to the first guest
NB *This will allow the walls, floor and benches to heat to the correct operating temperature*
4. Enter the Greek herbal bath and check the fibre optic lights are operating, and that the Greek herbal bath is clean and that all towels have been removed
5. Close the door to allow the room to reach its operating temperature
6. Check the temperature on the main control panel, this should be 60°C
(When switching on in the morning, it will take approximately 2 hours to reach this operating temperature)
7. Remove the herb trays, clean and replace
8. Place fresh herbs on the tray: chamomile, rosemary, lavender or salvia (sage)

Turkish hamman

Morning

1. Check the Turkish hamman is on – switch located in the plant room on the main control panel. Press the **green** button and the light will illuminate. This will turn on the heating
2. Turn on steam generator
3. Turn on the fibre optic lights
4. Turn on the Turkish hamman one hour prior to the first guest
NB *This will allow the walls, floor and benches to heat to the correct operating temperature*
5. Steam generation will commence once the correct temperature has been reached
6. Check the levels in the essence bottle and change if empty
NB *Unscrew and replace with new bottle of essence*
7. Enter the Turkish hamman and check the fibre optic lights are operating, that the Turkish hamman is clean and that all towels have been removed
8. Close the door to allow the room to reach its operating temperature
9. Check the temperature on the main control panel, this should be 60–80°C – ambient air temperature with steam
(When switching on in the morning, it will take approximately 2 hours to reach this temperature)

Morning Operations Instruction Sheet
By: Jane Crebbin-Bailey HCB Associates

Experience shower

Morning
1. Check the fibre optic lights are on
2. Check the levels of essence bottle and change if empty
   NB *Unscrew and replace with new bottle of essence*

Japanese salt bath

Morning
1. Check the Japanese salt bath is on. Switch located in the plant room on the main control panel. Press the **green** button and the light will illuminate. This will turn on the heating,
   NB *This will allow the walls, floor and benches to heat to the correct operating temperature*
2. Turn on the fibre optic lights
3. Check the levels in the essence bottle and change if empty
   NB *Unscrew and replace with new bottle of essence*
4. Enter the Japanese salt bath and check the fibre optic lights are operating, that the Japanese salt bath is clean and that all towels have been removed
5. Close the door to allow the room to reach its operating temperature
6. Check the temperature on the main control panel, this should be 45–48°C
   (When switching on in the morning, it will take approximately 2 hours to reach this operating temperature)
7. Wash the stones in the centre bowl with a suitable proprietary cleaning agent to remove any algae build-up

Tyrolean sauna

Morning
1. Check that the Tyrolean sauna has switched on automatically. If not, press start on the Tyrolean Sauna control panel – switch located in the plant room
2. Check that the Tyrolean sauna has been cleaned and that there are no towels left around

3. Check that the lights are on
4. Check that the floor mats (optional accessory) have been placed back into the Tyrolean sauna in the correct positions
5. Fill the bucket with water and ensure the ladle is to hand. Ladle 5 scoops of water on to the coals
6. The sauna will reach a temperature of 80–100°C within one hour
   NB *Please do not adjust the temperature settings without consulting the maintenance engineer*
   After 12 hours of continuous operating the Tyrolean sauna will automatically shut down
   NB *Should a longer period of operation be required, press the start button on the control panel in the plant room. The sauna will now operate for a further 12 hours. To stop the sauna during this period simply press the stop button on the control panel*

Laconium

Morning
1. Check the laconium is on. Switch located in the plant room on the main control panel
   Press the **green** button and the light will illuminate. This will turn on the heating
   NB *This will allow the walls, floor and benches to heat to the correct operating temperature*
2. Check the levels of essence bottle (orange essence) and change if empty
   NB *Unscrew and replace with new bottle of essence*
3. Enter the laconium and check the lights are operating, that the laconium is clean and that all towels have been removed
4. Close the door to allow the room to reach its operating temperature
5. Check the temperature on the main control panel, this should be 45–60°C, with 15–20 per cent humidity
   (When switching on in the morning, it will take approximately 2 hours to reach this operating temperature)

Evening Operations Instruction Sheet
By: Jane Crebbin-Bailey HCB Associates

Cleopatra slipper bath

Evening
To close down at night
1. Ensure the slipper bath is empty
2. Operate automatic disinfection programme (one hour)
3. Remove any towels, robes or paper cups
4. Extinguish the aromatic burner and candles
5. Clean the surface of the bath with a suitable non-abrasive proprietary cleaner
6. Ensure that the surrounding area is clean and dry
7. Leave the bath clean and dry overnight

Standard cleaning programme
The Cleopatra slipper bath should be cleaned with a suitable non-abrasive proprietary cleaner

Aqua meditation room

Evening
To close down at night
1. Ensure the aqua meditation room is empty
2. Press the **red** illuminated stop button – switch located in the plant room
3. Automatic draining and refilling of the water from the fountain and base of fountain
4. Remove any towels, robes or paper cups
5. Ensure the mirrored glass in fountain is clean
6. Check that the leather-style heated benches have been cleaned with a suitable proprietary cleaner to ensure hygiene standards are maintained
7. Turn off the music
8. Check the lights in the fountain are off
9. Ensure the floor is clean and any surface water is removed
10. Leave the door of the aqua meditation room open for 10 minutes and close upon leaving the spa

Standard cleaning programme
The aqua meditation room should be cleaned with sponges and a suitable proprietary cleaner

Indian blossom steam room

Evening
To close down at night
1. Ensure the Indian blossom steam room is empty
2. Press the **red** illuminated stop button – switch located in plant room
3. Remove any towels, robes or paper cups
4. Enter the Indian blossom steam room and spray the walls, benches and floor with the Kneipp hose
5. Check the fibre optic lighting is off
6. Leave the door open for 10 minutes and close upon leaving the spa

Standard cleaning programme
The Indian blossom steam room should be cleaned with a combination of bristle brushes on the mosaic surfaces and sponges for the tiles

NB *Deposits of calcium and scale may form on surfaces. A proprietary cleaning agent should be used each evening to avoid unsightly staining*

Evening Operations Instruction Sheet
By: Jane Crebbin-Bailey HCB Associates

Meditation room

Evening
1. Ensure the meditation room is empty
2. Extinguish the flame of the aromatic burner and empty the oil/water
3. Remove any discarded towels and paper cups from the meditation room
4. Check that the heating system is off by pressing the **red** illuminated stop button – located in the plant room

Standard cleaning programme
The ceramic heated couches should be cleaned with a combination of bristle brushes and sponges for the mosaic tiles

Reflexology footbaths

Evening
1. Ensure the reflexology basins are not in use
2. Remove any discarded towels and paper cups
3. Check the floor in the surrounding area is clean and any surface water is removed
4. Clean the basins and benches with a suitable disinfectant, to ensure hygiene standards are maintained
5. Check the heating system is off by turning lever to the right – located in the Plant room

Standard cleaning programme
The ceramic reflexology basins should be cleaned with a combination of bristle brushes and sponges for the mosaic tiles

Ice room

Evening
1. Ensure the ice room is empty
2. Remove any discarded towels and paper cups
3. Check the floor and surrounding area is clean and any surface water is removed
4. Clean the edge of the bowl and ledges of centre bowl
5. The ceramic reflexology basins should be cleaned with a combination of bristle brushes and sponges for the mosaic tiles
6. Close the door of the ice room to maintain the air-conditioned environment

Standard cleaning programme
The ceramic ice bowl should be cleaned with a combination of bristle brushes and sponges for the mosaic tiles.

Evening Operations Instruction Sheet
By: Jane Crebbin-Bailey HCB Associates

Serail

Evening
To close down the Serail at night
1. Ensure the serail is empty
2. Turn off the steam generator
3. Turn off the Serail
4. Turn off the fibre optic lights
5. Enter the Serail and spray the walls, benches and floor with the Kneipp hose
6. Ensure that all mud containers are sealed and that the stock levels are monitored

Standard cleaning programme
The Serail should be cleaned with a combination of bristle brushes on the mosaic surfaces and sponges for the tiles

NB *Because steam is generated in the Serail, deposits of calcium and scale may form on surfaces, especially at the base of the steam inlet. A proprietary cleaning agent should be used each evening to avoid unsightly staining*

Greek herbal bath

Evening
To close down at night and commence the automatic disinfecting routine
1. Ensure the Greek herbal bath is empty
2. Press the **red** illuminated stop button – located in the plant room
3. Enter the Greek herbal bath and spray the walls, benches and floor with the Kneipp hose
4. Press the 'disinfecting' button – located in the plant room
   Automatic cleaning cycle: the walls, benches and floor will now heat up to a temperature of 80°C to kill off any bacteria. This process takes 40 minutes and will shut off automatically
5. Leave the door open for 10 minutes and close upon leaving the spa
   NB *Do not enter the Greek herbal bath during this time*

Standard cleaning programme
The Greek herbal bath should be cleaned with a combination of bristle brushes on the mosaic surfaces and sponges for the tiles

NB *Because steam is generated in the Greek herbal bath, deposits of calcium and scale may form on surfaces, especially at the base of the steam inlet. A proprietary cleaning agent should be used each evening to avoid unsightly staining*

Turkish hamman

Evening
To close down the Turkish hamman at night
1. Ensure the Turkish hamman is empty
2. Check that the heating system is off by pressing the **red** illuminated stop button – located in the plant room
3. Turn off the steam generator
4. Turn off the fibre optic lights
5. Enter the Turkish hamman and spray the walls, benches and floor with the Kneipp hose
6. Leave the door open for 10 minutes and close upon leaving the spa

Standard cleaning programme
The Turkish hamman should be cleaned with a combination of bristle brushes on the mosaic surfaces and sponges for the tiles

NB *Because steam is generated in the Turkish hamman, deposits of calcium and scale may form on surfaces, especially at the base of the steam inlet. A proprietary cleaning agent should be used each evening to avoid unsightly staining*

Evening Operations Instruction Sheet
By: Jane Crebbin-Bailey HCB Associates

The experience shower

Evening
To close down at night
1. Ensure the showers are empty and clean

Standard cleaning programme
The showers should be cleaned with a combination of bristle brushes on the mosaic surfaces and sponges for the tiles

NB *Because steam is generated in the experience showers, deposits of calcium and scale may form on surfaces, especially at the base of the steam inlet. A proprietary cleaning agent should be used each evening to avoid unsightly staining*

Japanese salt bath

Evening
To close down at night
1. Ensure the Japanese salt bath is empty
2. Press the **red** illuminated stop button – located in the plant room
3. Enter the Japanese salt bath, spray the walls, benches and floor with the Kneipp hose
4. Leave the door open for 10 minutes and close upon leaving the spa

Standard cleaning programme
The Japanese salt bath should be cleaned with a combination of bristle brushes on the mosaic surfaces and sponges for the tiles

Wash the stones in the centre bowl with a suitable proprietary cleaning agent to remove any algae build-up

NB *Because salt steam is generated in the Japanese salt bath, deposits of calcium and scale may form on surfaces, especially at the base of the steam inlet. A proprietary cleaning agent should be used each evening to avoid unsightly staining*

Tyrolean sauna

Evening
To close down at night
1. At the end of the day ensure that the Tyrolean sauna has either switched off automatically or press the **red** stop button on the control panel
2. Open the Tyrolean sauna door
3. Clean the floor and benches with a suitable disinfectant
4. Leave the Tyrolean sauna door open during the night to ensure that the sauna can dry out
   NB *This is essential for the preservation of the timber*

LACONIUM

Evening
To close down at night
1. Ensure the laconium is empty
2. Press the **red** illuminated stop button – located in the plant room
3. Enter the laconium and spray the walls, benches and floor with the Kneipp hose
4. Leave the door open for 10 minutes and close upon leaving the spa

Standard cleaning programme
The laconium should be cleaned with a combination of bristle brushes on the mosaic surfaces and sponges for the tiles

Wash the stones in the centre bowl with a suitable proprietary cleaning agent to remove any algae build-up

NB *Deposits of calcium and scale may form on surfaces. A proprietary cleaning agent should be used each evening to avoid unsightly staining*

Morning/Evening Operations Instruction Sheet
By: Jane Crebbin-Bailey HCB Associates

Ice fountain

Morning
1. Check the ice fountain is producing ice
2. Remove any discarded towels and paper cups
3. Check the floor in the surrounding area is clean and any surface water is removed
4. Check the temperature. This should be 15°C
5. Break up the ice in the centre bowl
6. Clean edge of bowl and ledges of centre bowl
7. Check that the ice release sensors are not blocked

Ice fountain

Evening
1. Remove any discarded towels and paper cups
2. Check the floor and surrounding area is clean and any surface water is removed
3. Clean the edge of bowl and lion's head entrance.
4. Check that the ice sensors are not blocked with ice
5. The ceramic surround should be cleaned with a combination of bristle brushes and sponges for the mosaic tiles

Standard cleaning programme
The ceramic ice bowl should be cleaned with a combination of bristle brushes and sponges for the mosaic tiles.

References

Health and Safety Executive, 1999, *Managing Health and Safety in Swimming Pools,* HSG179, HSE Books, London.

Health and Safety Executive, 2000, *Legionnaires' Disease – the Control of Legionella Bacteria in Water Systems*, 3rd edn, L8, HSE Books, London.

Health and Safety Executive, 2002, *Legionnaire's Disease, Approved Code of Practice and Guidance.* Health & Safety Executive Books, London.

Jokinen, E., I. Valimaki, K. Antila, Sepponen, A. and Tuomina, J., 1990, 'Children in sauna: Cardiovascular adjustment', *Pediatrics*, 86/2, 282–7.

Pool Water Treatment Advisory Group, 1999, *Swimming Pool Water, Treatment and Quality Standards*, Pool Water Treatment Advisory Group, Norfolk.

Press, E., 1991, 'The health hazards of saunas and spas and how to minimise them', *American Journal of Public Health*, 81/8, 1034–7.

Public Health Laboratory, *Hygiene for Spa Pools*, Public Health Laboratory, PHLS Water Environmental Microbiology, London.

Shinaberger, C.S., Anderson, C.L. and Kraus, J.F., 1990, 'Young children who drown in hot tubs and whirlpools in California: A 26-year study', *American Journal of Public Health*, 80/5, 613–14.

St John Ambulance, St Andrews Ambulance Association and the Red Cross, 2002, *First Aid Manual*, 8th edn, St John Ambulance, St Andrews Ambulance Association and the Red Cross, United Kingdom.

Useful addresses

Pool Water Treatment Advisory Group, www.pwtag.demon.co.uk

Swimming Pool and Allied Trades Association (SPATA), www.spata.co.uk

The Hydrotherapy Association Advice Centre, PO Box 30, Godalming, Surrey GU7 1LG.

The mind–body connection

6

The effect of the mind over the body

Philosophers have argued for centuries over the concept of the mind. More recently neurophysiologists and neuropharmacologists have joined in the debate. The mind can be defined as the functions in an individual person dealing with feelings, perception, thoughts, willpower and reason.

As shown in Chapter 1, medicine and magic were intertwined up to the time of Hippocrates (c.450–370 BC), when his followers rejected the supernatural theories and promoted the idea of disease being due to the imbalance of humours or fluids in the body. Plato (427–347 BC) was the first to disagree with this, maintaining that it was a mistake to separate the soul from the body. However, the humoral theory of health depending on the balance of natural substances in the body was perpetuated by Galen of Pergamum and although altered by anatomical and pathological discoveries from the sixteenth century onwards, the idea has influenced western medicine in different forms until the twentieth century.

In other cultures, such as Ayurvedic and traditional Chinese medicine, imbalance as the cause of ill health underlies many philosophies – see the sections on alternate and energy medicines in Chapter 4.

What is the evidence for the mind–body connection? The 'mind–body' interface has been the subject of much discussion and research in recent years. At present, brain chemistry appears to be the link between the mind and the body. Two types of chemical are involved:-

Neuropeptides

An endogenous peptide (a chemical obtained from the partial hydrolysis of proteins within the body) for example an endorphin or an encephalin that influences neural activity or functioning. In the 1970s, naturally occurring painkillers whose structure resembled morphine were discovered. They were called 'endorphins' – short for endogenous morphine or body-produced morphine. There is now a considerable mass of evidence to support the theory that placebos trigger the release of endorphins via the brain's pituitary and hypothalamus glands to decrease pain, but the mechanism for this is still obscure.

Neurotransmitters

Chemical messengers released from a nerve ending when a nerve impulse arrives and interacts with an adjacent nerve, muscle fibre or gland to produce an inhibitory or excitatory response. Examples of neurotransmitters are adrenaline and noradrenaline, the endorphins and seratonin.

Psychosomatic illness

This is an illness related to stress, for example migraine, indigestion, asthma or gastric ulcer,

The power of suggestion

This is the interaction between the psyche and the functioning of the body in order to harness the will and energy of the patient in order to aid and release the self-healing capabilities of the person. This is part of the placebo response.

Placebo effect

Surveys have showed that a proportion of the improvement in an illness is due to four factors:

1. the environment in which treatment is received

2. the relationship between patient and practitioner

3. the way in which the illness is explained and approached by the therapist

4. healing as a result of belief in the treatment.

The consequences of these factors, apart from the impact of the medication or procedures themselves, is called 'the placebo effect'. This is separate from the spontaneous cures and the natural remissions which occur in some illnesses. Recovery also depends on a number of other factors including the natural progression of the disease and the extent of the immune response.

The meaning of placebo comes from the Latin, 'I please', suggesting that the result brings pleasure to the recipient and that the effect also occurs to please an outsider, for example a therapist or relative. Therefore the placebo effect is the proportion of the improvement in the condition of a sick person, which cannot be considered to be due to the specific treatment employed. Recent research has indicated that this phenomenon is due to changes in neuropeptides in the brain which control stress and relieve pain. These chemicals are also released at acupuncture sites.

The proportion of improvement in an illness attributable to the placebo effect varies due to the factors already described. However, it can be as high as 30 per cent and change from person to person.

Good clinical trials are now designed to take this into account, by comparing those having no treatment with active and placebo groups.

The belief effect

The effectiveness of a placebo is dependent on the extent of the belief of the patient. Time spent with the patient, a sympathetic practitioner or the strength of therapist authority, for example the 'white coat' factor plus the effect of technology – a black box or a shining, humming machine – only produce the effect indirectly, by altering or reinforcing the beliefs of the patient.

Placebos only seem to work as much as the patient believes they will; the more credible they seem, the greater the effect. The result of the placebo will differ from person to person. What works for one may not work for another and this might explain the variations seen in clinical trials. To this must be added the fact that not all illnesses respond to placebos.

The pathogenesis of psychosomatic illness

Changes in the environment or threats to a human being, such as fear, apprehension and insecurity, cause a reaction to protect the body by activating the defence mechanisms. This occurs via the sympathetic nervous system. The hypothalamus and pituitary glands in the brain programme the adrenal glands to release adrenaline and steroid hormones. Production of endorphins is also monitored by these two glands.

The mobilisation of these 'fight or flight' mechanisms of the body's defences is far reaching and affects breathing, digestion, the heart, the blood circulation, the metabolism, the mind and even alters muscle action. The emotions are functions from earlier evolutionary development to enable humans to marshal all their defence mechanisms quickly.

Nowadays, there are many situations where 'fight or flight' responses are inappropriate. A continuous state of reaction to stress and threat results in the over-arousal of these reactions, which may lead to the physical impairment of function in the body systems affected.

Over-stimulation may result in gastric ulceration, breathing difficulties, high blood pressure, fatigue, irritability, headaches and migraine. One of the most important effects is the weakening of the immune function and the lowering of the body's resistance to disease when under strain.

To counteract this, the secret is to switch off from stress, but this is easier said than done. So often, stress becomes a chronic or persistent phenomenon in certain types of personality.

Spas and the placebo

Spas are usually situated in quiet, beautiful surroundings and are invariably impressively designed, decorated and appointed. The relaxing spa environment is a complete change from the everyday stresses and strains of life. This enables the body to 'switch off' and lessen the 'fight or flight' responses.

Many spas, especially those on the continent, claim several centuries of healing, encouraging clients to book and arrive in the belief that they will benefit from the experience. These factors, in addition to the relationship between therapist and client, 'the white coat factor' of the practitioner and unusual, different spa treatments all contribute to the placebo effect. This is not to say that spas only work through the placebo response.

Because spas are primarily places of relaxation and tension release, they help many conditions, especially those which are stress-related. Treatments are non-invasive and relatively safe, with no serious side effects.

The minimum effect spas can achieve is to lift the spirit, enhance the 'feel-good' factor and enable the client to manage their disability or problem in a more positive way. Usually, much more is attained (see below).

The psychology of bathing and spas

Everyone starts life surrounded by water: a baby's development begins in water; this is the amniotic fluid surrounds it from conception to birth. The developing foetus spends the first nine months of its life getting ready for the big, wide world in air. When someone takes a bath or spa treatment, immersion in water recalls our past. Many people feel 'at home' in water.

Subconsciously, those first nine months surrounded by amniotic fluid leave a life-long impression. When in water, the psyche is reminded of the safety, security and comfort of the womb. This makes bathing such a restorative experience. Immersion in water is also a soothing sensation. There is, however, much more to bathing than the feeling of being cocooned in the past.

The power of culture

The power of bathing is rooted in our culture, together with the spa concept. The belief in the healing power of water goes back to the earliest of civilisations and the days of magic and medicine. Bathing and religious purification and healing went hand in hand for centuries (see Chapter 1).

Spas have a long history of healing, stretching back many centuries. Clients visit a spa or undergo water treatment expecting to feel better, to stave off disease or to obtain some help to fight an illness in the belief that they will become healthier.

The factors involved

There are very few research papers on the psychology of immersion. The reason for the improvement of mood after bathing is known to be complex and due to many different factors. By looking at the many and varied changes which take place on water immersion, some of the reasons for this 'feel-good factor' can be appreciated.

Feeling buoyed up

Psychological change is brought about by the physical effects of immersion, which are mainly due to buoyancy or the capacity to float in water. (This is discussed in Chapter 2.) The ability to float depends on the density of the water or quantity of minerals dissolved in it. In the most dense water – Droitwich brine or the Dead Sea – floating is easy and we experience almost complete weightlessness, allowing the body to relax to varying degrees. There is some buoyancy in ordinary tap water, but it is not so marked as in more heavily mineralised water.

When immersed in dense water, the human frame feels as if it has been released from a straitjacket. Joints and muscles move more easily in water than on land and this is proportional to the density. The downward and depressing effect of gravity is reduced and countered by an upward and equal force, as stated in Archimedes' Principle (see Chapter 2). For a time afterwards, the client feels like a different person – lighter and less weighed down by the cares of the world, having experienced a partial decrease in the gravitational load. For the same reason, movements in joints and muscles seem easier. Release from the constant effects of gravity produces a feeling of elation, euphoria and being buoyed up.

Changes in body image

As well as feeling lighter in water, people perceive themselves to be smaller, more lithe and lissom. Standing in a swimming pool and looking down at ourselves, the body appears to have shrunk in water – the body image changes and for the better. Researchers have shown that a woman standing up to her breastbone in water only 'sees' or experiences 28 per cent of her body weight. She feels less heavy, more graceful – a different woman, in fact, as indeed she is for that moment of time.

Immersion changes the amounts of the anti-diuretic hormone which controls urine production (see Chapter 2, page 42 on renal effects). As a result, urine output increases up to six-fold, depending on the length of immersion, and most spa users know that the kidneys remove waste products and toxins and so, mentally, they feel cleansed and detoxified by this outflow.

Hydrostatic pressure, the pressure exerted by the water surrounding the body, reduces the amount of fluid in waterlogged tissues – called oedema – especially around the joints and lower legs. As a result, there is weight loss and again the perception of the body image improves. Joints are easier to move because of the loss of fluid, which enables more freedom of movement and flexibility.

In addition, skin texture is changed – often feeling softer and suppler. All these factors contribute to a positive alteration in body image.

The effect of temperature

Another factor in the psychology of water is the temperature at which it is experienced. In water at body temperature – termed thermoneutral – hormonal changes are triggered by the pituitary gland in the brain. One of these changes liberates ACTH (adrenocorticotrophic hormone). This, in turn, prompts the production of corticosteroids from the adrenal glands situated on the top of each kidney. One of these is cortisol, otherwise known as hydrocortisone, used in medical creams as an anti-inflammatory agent. It also regulates glucose and protein metabolism, the immune response in the body and alters the reaction to stress. It also imparts to the brain a sense of euphoria and well-being.

Hot water – above body temperature (37°C) – encourages blood to go to the skin and muscles. The improved blood supply removes waste products such as lactic acid, which contribute to muscle aches and pains. Warm stimulation of thermo-receptors in the skin relaxes stretch receptors in muscles to relieve tension and allay anxiety in these soft tissues. The result is that we feel more comfortable, secure and soothed.

Cold water (around 18°C) has benefits too. The circulation in the skin shuts down and blood is shunted into the heart, main blood vessels within the chest cavity and carotid arteries taking blood to the brain. The latter dilate to accommodate the increase in blood volume and, as a result of the improved brain perfusion, the person feels more alert and lively. In addition, cold water acts as an analgesic to deaden pain and this also contributes to the experience of euphoria.

Stimulation of the five senses

Spas stimulate the five senses in the following ways:

- *Sight* The sight of water is relaxing. Reflections and moving water are fascinating. The spa environment

– lighting, the glow of candles, the many hues of floating flower petals, or the colours of the water and the décor of the surroundings all play a vital role in the pleasant and soothing experience of bathing.

- *Sound* The swish and murmur of moving water when swimming, or the rustle of air through jets in water and the burble of bubbles – all these sounds are calming and comforting.

- *Smell* Additives such as essential oils give off odours, which can stimulate or relax both mind and body. The smell of algae and seaweed recall trips to the sea and the sight and sound of roaring waves on the shore. The sea air is perceived to be bracing, fresh and clean.

- *Taste* A glass of water before and after treatment is refreshing and imparts a sense of cleanliness to the regime, in addition to countering any degree of dehydration, which imparts a below par feeling.

- *Touch* Being enveloped in and surrounded by water is comforting and adds a sense of security. There are, again, echoes of the womb. Additives not only stimulate the sense of smell, they make the skin feel different.

Oils, algae, seaweed and the minerals in thermal waters and brine, or the Dead Sea, all play their part in changing the perception of the body image. These additives have a tonic effect on the skin and impart a soft, silky feel, which is extremely pleasant. Additives serve as a tangible reminder and reinforce the belief that water is of benefit to the body.

The part played by massage

Massage by jet or human hands adds its own particular dimension to the treatment and to the pleasurable sensations of the spa experience. The skin and soft tissues are caressed, easing away toxins and tensions. Massage techniques are very personal and, being a one-to-one situation, the client feels 'special', with a treatment tailored for them.

Touch has healing powers of its own, especially in the hands of an expert. Healers and the healed down the ages have had faith in 'the laying on of hands'.

Positive and negative ions

The 'feel good factor' also owes something to ions in the atmosphere (see Chapter 3. Uses of Water – pages 49–51).

These various stimuli enhance the special event of bathing and spa attendance, producing changes in the psyche that make clients feel different and feel better. Such is the psychology behind the spa experience.

References

Bynum, W.F. and Roy Porter (eds), 1993, *Companion Encyclopedia of the History of Medicine*, Routledge, London.

Campion, Margaret Reid, 1997, *Hydrotherapy, Principles and Practice*, Butterworth Heinemann, London.

Evans, Dylan, 2003, *Placebo, the Belief Effect*, HarperCollins, London.

Fulder, Stephen, 1988, *The Handbook of Complementary Medicine*, Oxford University Press, Oxford.

Holford, Patrick and Hyla Cass, 2001, *Natural Highs*, Piatkus, London.

Levine, J.D., N.C. Gordon *et al*, 1978, 'The mechanism of placebo analgesia', *The Lancet*, 2, 654–7.

Readers Digest, 1991, *The Readers Digest Family Guide to Alternative Medicine*, Readers Digest Association.

Webster's Medical Desk Dictionary, 1988, Merriam-Webster Inc.

Zollman, C. and A. Vickers, 2000, *The ABC of Complementary Medicine*, BMJ Publications.

The way ahead

7

Despite its long and exciting history, spa in its present form is a relatively new business. Spa as a descriptive noun in its current usage describes a place for relaxation, revitalisation, spiritual awareness, physical well-being (a fit mind in a fit body) and pampering. A spa is a place where, through design and targeted management action, people are encouraged to develop awareness of both the spiritual and physical factors which effect, and benefit, their feeling of well-being.

The first known use of the word spa is by the Romans 'Salus Par Aqua' – health through water. This is the name given by the Romans to the first known Roman baths in Northern Europe – Spa in Belgium – a name that was taken by the town that grew up around the Roman baths.

Legend has it that the wife of a Roman military leader during the Northern campaign, probably around 50–100 AD, became ill and was cured at the place we now know as Spa in Belgium. Word spread and from that time on that name, Spa, was given to all the places that had thermal water springs – Bath in the UK, Baden-Baden in Germany, Budapest in Hungary, Gerona on the Iberian peninsular and many others.

In Roman times the spa was where people met to converse, to philosophise, and to discuss politics and the happenings of the day in a relaxed atmosphere. They were the centres of social life for soldiers and administrators. The Romans built spas all over Europe, wherever indigenous water sources were found. The most famous of these, and the best preserved, is in the City of Bath 120 miles west of London – although Baden-Baden in Germany runs a pretty close second.

The Roman baths in Gerona on the Iberian Peninsular, which were later rebuilt and used by the Arab occupiers in the twelfth century – hence the remains are now called 'The Roman-Arabische Baths' – show how these baths were constructed by Roman engineers to provide a sequence of heat experiences for the spa goer.

As you enter, the first room is the antedarium, which we would call a changing room, the next is the tepidarium, which is warm and relaxing, the next is the laconium, which is a dry heat – hotter than the tepidarium – and the third is the caldarium, which is very hot and humid – almost like a Turkish bath today. Next to the caldarium was the fire chamber, which heated water to be circulated, by gravity, beneath the floors of the adjoining 'spa rooms'. This was the first known use of underfloor heating in the modern world, over 2000 years ago.

As the water progressed under the floor of the chambers, it gradually cooled, hence the progression of spa experiences from hot and steamy in the caldarium to a warm relaxing heat in the tepidarium, with the laconium, a dry heat like a sauna, in the middle. The water was then pumped, by a paddle wheel operated manually (no doubt by slaves) back to the tank above the fire chamber (read treatment card 'The Use and Application of the Thermarium Tepidarium/Meditation Room').

The baths in those far-off days were the centre of the community, the place where people met. Later, after the Dark Ages, from the sixteenth to the early twentieth centuries, when religions flourished, churches took over this role in society. More recently, in the middle to the latter part of the twentieth century, pubs (public houses that sell alcohol in the UK and Ireland), coffee houses and cafés became the social centres of communities.

Today, more people meet their future husbands or wives either at work, or at a sports or fitness club, than anywhere else. Things would appear to have come full circle as in the twenty-first century, sports and fitness clubs – which are metamorphosing into spas – fulfil the cultural, social and philosophical role in society started by the Romans in the first century AD.

So, where are spas going in the twenty-first century? 'I would expect that spas in the future will encompass two diverse trends', claims Suzanne Ng, Spa Director of The Spa at The Mandarin Oriental, New York. 'One will be more medically concentrated with the focus on anti-ageing medical programmes and techniques with a much more

The Use and Application of the Thermarium
Tepidarium/Meditation Room

By: Jane Crebbin-Bailey HCB Associates

Benefit of treatment

This room consists of a relaxation area with ergonomic heated ceramic couches. You can stay in this room for long periods to relax. The heated ceramic couches warm up your body which is ideal prior to massage treatments or also (or between) the other heat experiences.

Advantages

- The temperature operates between 42–45°C – ambient air temperature
- Fully-tiled heated walls, floor and ergonomic heated ceramic couches – 6 persons
- Painted walls
- Emergency call button

Contra-indications and precautions

- Cardiovascular disease (heart failure, coronary disease, strokes)
- Respiratory disease – severe asthma requiring regular inhaler use
- Client feels unwell with a fever
- High/low blood pressure
- Infected skin wounds
- Uncontrolled epilepsy

Preparation

- Operator/reception – First part of the day – Turn on system as per manufacturer's instructions (see 'Daily Operating Instructions Card')

Method

The tepidarium should be included as part of a sequence:

- Relax on your towel on the heated ceramic couches
- Rest for 20 minutes before either returning to the caldarium, laconium, hydro pool or other treatment involved in a sequence
- Shower after the meditation room with cold or warm water

After care

- Rest for about 20 minutes, preferably in a warm gown on a recliner
- Drink several glasses of water
- Apply a good moisturiser to the skin after a shower or follow on with another treatment

Maintenance

- Read 'Daily Operating Instructions Card'
- Clean seating area of the ceramic heated couches with a disinfectant suitable for ceramic tiles
- Check cleanliness of area on a regular basis – towels, floor, seating area, etc.
- Check level of essence in the aromatic burners or aromatic candles

www.spa-therapy.com

©HCB Associates   Mar 2001

clinical and scientific approach. The other, which will be the way for the most exclusive spas, will be "temples" where holistic wellness is lived and breathed, incorporating all the holistic healing elements of the East and West, becoming lifestyle places where education and therapy are one and the same' (*Pulse Magazine*, August 2003, pp 14–16).

Types of spa

Day spa

Day spas are generally targeted at the city dweller with limited leisure time. They provide an oasis of tranquillity and peace in a busy urban location. The facilities visitors can expect from this type of spa are:

- cloakroom or lockers (for storing clients outdoor wear)
- a variety of facial and body treatments including massage techniques
- private treatment rooms for each client receiving a personal service with shower facilities
- professional, fully-trained therapists and specialist staff holding recognised national qualifications
- a range of complementary homecare products
- detailed full-day and half-day spa programmes
- rest and relaxation area
- bathrobes, towels and slippers provided, where applicable
- a consultation/health check on their first visit

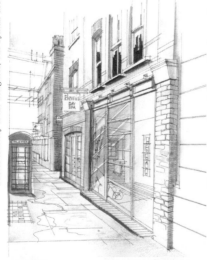

Photos courtesy of the designers, The Syntax Group

The Elemis Day Spa, Mayfair, London, UK

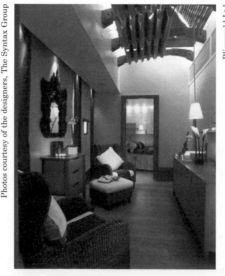

Photos courtesy of the designers, The Syntax Group

A double treatment suite at The Elemis Day Spa
www.elemis.com

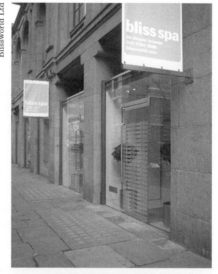

Blissworld Ltd

Bliss Spa, London, UK
www.bliss.com

and one or more of the following:

- hydrotherapy
- water-based treatments
- steam treatments
- spa cuisine
- fitness facility
- nutrition and weight management
- experience showers
- dedicated changing rooms.

Destination spa

A destination spa's sole purpose is to provide guests with lifestyle improvement and health enhancement through professionally administered spa services, physical fitness, educational programming and on-site accommodation. Spa cuisine is served exclusively.

The facilities should include:

- tranquil and/or spectacular location
- landscaped gardens or parkland
- healthy food catering for specialist diets – spa cuisine
- nutrition and weight management
- daily activities programmes geared to fitness and health
- outdoor activities
- a variety of facial and body treatments, including massage techniques, provided with qualified on-site medical supervision

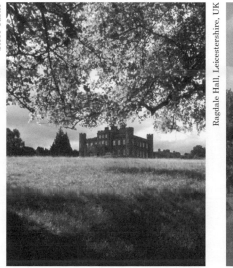

Stobo Castle, Peebles, Scotland   **Ragdale Hall, Leicestershire, UK**

- a variety of alternative/complementary therapies
- hairdressing, make-over, manicure and pedicure facilities
- private treatment rooms for each client receiving a personal service with shower facilities
- professional, fully-trained therapists and specialist staff with recognised national qualifications
- health check at the beginning of their stay
- detailed spa programmes
- a range of complementary homecare products
- seeks to educate its guests through talks/lectures and lifestyle-enhancing programmes
- indoor/outdoor swimming pool for relaxation
- water-based spa treatments
- rest and relaxation common areas
- supervised fitness facility/gym
- complementary bathrobe, towels and slippers.

Medical spa

This category includes individuals, solo practices, groups and institutions whose primary purpose is to provide comprehensive medical and wellness care in an environment which integrates spa services, as well as conventional and complimentary therapies and treatments.

Mineral spring spa

This is a spa offering an on-site source of mineral, thermal or seawater used in hydrotherapy treatments. Often there

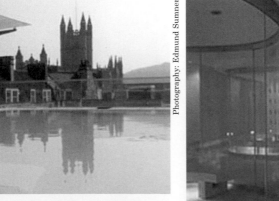

The roof top thermal pool at Thermae Bath Spa, Bath, Somerset, UK

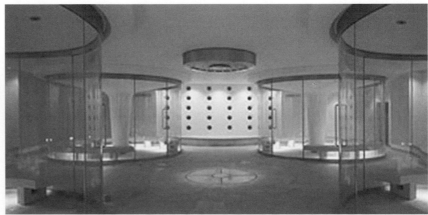

Steam pods, with cenral drench shower, at The Thermae Bath Spa, Bath, Somerset, UK

is an overlap between medical spas and mineral spring spas, as they both tend to use the water for its curative properties. However, you don't need to have an ailment to visit a mineral spring spa. You may want to take the water purely for relaxation, or to enhance your well-being by taking preventative measures against disease. Europe is well-known for its hot mineral springs.

Resort or hotel

A spa owned by, and located within, a resort or hotel providing professionally administered spa services, fitness and well-being components and spa cuisine menu choices. In addition to the leisure guest, this is a great place for business travellers who wish to take advantage of the spa experience while away from home. They are frequently an oasis of tranquillity and peace located within, or adjacent to a 4- or 5-star hotel, whether town centre or resort. They provide relaxation and escape from a busy schedule for the discerning traveller.

Resort spas have the following facilities:

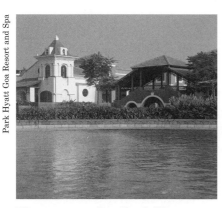

The spectacular Park Hyatt Resort and Spa, in Goa, one of the first true resort spas on the Indian sub-continent

- cloakrooms (for storing clients' outdoor wear)
- a variety of facial and body treatments including massage techniques
- private treatment rooms for each client receiving a personal service with shower facilities
- professional, fully-trained therapists and specialist staff holding recognised national qualifications
- a range of complementary homecare products
- detailed full-day and half-day spa programs
- rest and relaxation area
- bathrobes, towels and slippers provided, where applicable
- healthy foods catering for specialist diets in the hotel
- a fitness facility/gym and swimming pool

and one or more of the following:

- hydrotherapy
- water-based treatments
- steam treatments
- nutrition and weight management
- experience showers
- dedicated changing rooms.

Park Hyatt Goa Resort and Spa

Spa design and operations

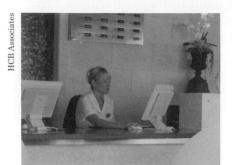

HCB Associates

**Reception, Le Spa at
Le Meridien, Cyprus**

HCB Associates

**Reception area, Chapel Spa,
Cheltenham, UK**

Design is by its nature subjective. A design that one person likes or considers good and functional will be deplored by others as fussy and unimaginative. Design is subject to trends and the foibles of fashion and is constantly evolving.

Design is an expression of function. Therefore, with spa design we need to specify the functions or individual areas of the spa. These can be simply divided into wet areas and dry areas, which should as far as possible be kept apart.

- Dry areas: Reception
  Relaxation area
  Dry treatment rooms
  Staff and management facilities
- Wet areas: Changing areas, including showers
  Kitchens
  Pools
  Wet treatment suites, including massage

Relaxation area

The hub of all spa operations should be the relaxation area. Clients list relaxation as the main reason for visiting a spa. Therefore, this is the area which has the most importance as the client will spend more conscious time here than anywhere else in the spa.

The relaxation area or facility, where there is space, may well be both inside and outside. Even in small buildings in towns and cities, a light well or roof space can be adapted for use as a part of the relaxation facility for the client. A relaxation area in a spa is more that just a room or area with a couple of loungers and soft lights. It should be a quiet area, with a focal point, and treat the five senses (see Chapter 4, page 119 and Chapter 6, page 191).

Reception

The reception area is obviously very important, as this is the first impression that the client will get. The function of the reception area is to present the spa's offering to the world. Therefore the design must reflect this. There are some common errors in creating reception areas:

- Insufficient stations – a receptionist should be nothing else. Nothing annoys a new client more than

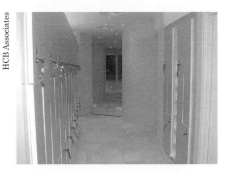

Locker Room, Spa Changing Rooms at Chewton Glen Hotel & Spa, Hampshire, UK

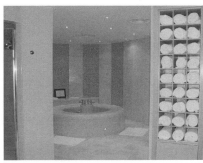

Locker Room, Spa Changing Rooms at Chewton Glen Hotel & Spa, Hampshire, UK. Designed by HCB Associates

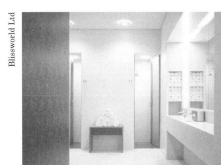

Locker Room, Bliss, London

waiting at a reception desk while the receptionist answers the telephone. Ideally there should be three stations: one for a receptionist who greets the client, a second for a telephonist/scheduler who answers the telephone and takes bookings and a third for a spa hostess/guide, who can explain all treatments and procedures and show the client where to go and what to do.

● Chairs for clients waiting – unless absolutely unavoidable never put waiting chairs in the reception area, clients should wait in the relaxation area – starting their spa experience as soon as possible after entering the spa.

Changing rooms

Changing rooms are another misunderstood opportunity. Too many spas use these as simply places for clients to change! Ideally the client, when in the spa, should be wearing spa wear provided by the spa, whether gowns, track suits, kimonos, sarongs or bespoke designed spa outfits. These are handed to the client by the spa hostess/guide at the reception.

On entry into the changing room, the client will shower and change into the spa wear. The changing room should have a theme which reflects the philosophy of the spa. As an example, one spa in India has a poem as the theme in the changing area:

LOOK TO THIS DAY

Look to this day
For it is Life
The very Life of Life
In its brief course lie all
The realities and truths of existence
The joy of growth
The splendour of action
The glory of power
For yesterday is but a memory
And tomorrow is only a vision
But today well lived
Makes every yesterday a memory of happiness
And every tomorrow a vision of hope
Look well therefore to this day.

KALIDASA
(Indian poet and playwright – probably second or third century)

Where possible, the changing room should lead straight from the reception, and proceed through to the relaxation area. Therefore, the spa hostess/guide can then show the client, with their spa wear, the changing room and the relaxation room. The spa hostess can explain all of the facilities in both the changing room and the relaxation area. They can inform the client that they will be collected by their therapist if they are having treatments or explain to the client the rest of the facilities within the spa, such as steam or heat, which may be available.

The relaxation area should be located adjacent to the wet and dry treatment areas. The spa therapists can then collect their clients for their scheduled appointments.

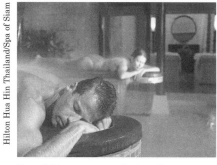

Dual Treatment Suite Hyatt Hua Hin, Thailand

Treatment rooms

The revenue producing areas of the spa are the treatment rooms and facilities, most of which are covered in earlier sections of this book. In the ideal spa layout, the relaxation room might lead into a corridor with the wet spa areas at one end and the dry treatment rooms at the other or even be placed between the two.

The trend today is toward double treatment suites. Many people visit spas as couples or pairs and naturally want to have treatments together. It is even sometimes daunting to be shut in a room with a therapist you do not know, lying on a couch, naked, feeling very vulnerable. Double treatment suites can be two treatment areas, perhaps linked by a dedicated relaxation space, with a treatment couch in one part and a facial chair or piece of equipment such as a hydrotherapy bath or dry float bed in the other. The spa will perhaps market treatments or packages for couples – husband and wife, mother and daughter, or just two friends – whilst one is having a hydrotherapy treatment the other can be having a massage.

When considering space allocation, a treatment room should be no smaller than 2m × 4m or 8m^2 and a double treatment suite 4m × 8m or 32m^2. Space will also need to be allocated for staff rooms and management offices, laundry and housekeeping services.

Spa cuisine

A light spa cuisine lunch is frequently included, sometimes bought in from a nearby café or prepared in the spa's own kitchen, and served in the relaxation area. All the consultations between therapist and client are carried out in the treatment suite.

General interest

The popularity of spas around the world today is evidenced by the proliferation of spa books, magazines and articles in general interest news media. Every major title today has a spa, well-being or lifestyle editor, dedicated primarily to reporting on happenings in the spa world, in day spas, resort/hotel spas or destination spas from Sydney to New York, St. Petersburg to Cape Town, and everywhere in between.

Industry research

Research has been carried out in the US by FO Plog Research for the International Spa Association (www.experienceispa.com). This reported that 21 per cent of the US population visited at least one type of spa in the 12 months up to June 2003 and that on average spa-goers visit 2 spas per year.

In the UK research by Allegra Strategies (www.allegra.co.uk) indicates dynamic growth fuelled by increasing consumer demand, with revenue increasing by 11 per cent year-on-year and the number of outlets growing by 8 per cent each year.

Australia

In Australia, research by Singapore-based Intelligent Spas Pty. Ltd for the Australasian Spa Association (www.intelligentspas.com) shows that, although starting from a lower base, the growth of the Australasian market is equally dramatic with 220 spas employing more than 3000 people and generating $15 million revenue (£6.5 million) in 2002.

United States

The Plog US survey was carried out online on 14–19 June, 2003 with 1201 respondents. 'Three hundred surveys were completed in Canada, the UK and Japan regarding spa visitation,' Scott Ludwigsen of Pheonix Marketing International told the delegates. 'The propensity of spa visitation is higher in each of these countries than the US; more than half of the people in the UK and Japan report visiting a spa in the past twelve months,' he said.

In the US more than 44 million individual visits were made during the year, with 25.6 million visits recorded to day spas; 16 million to resort/hotel spas and only 2.2 million to destination spas. Medical spas and mineral spring spas exceeded destination spa visits with more than 4 million recorded for each. These numbers should be considered against the US national census which shows that there are 224.7 million people aged 16+ in the US.

Massage was the most popular treatment with 70 per cent of respondents indicating this as their preference. Facials, manicures and steam baths were also shown to be popular. The figure of 70 per cent shows a marked increase on a similar survey carried out by PriceWaterhouseCoopers for ISPA in 2002 in which massage was reported to produce 49 per cent of treatment room revenue with facials producing 39 per cent and wet treatments 15 per cent.

United Kingdom

The UK study by Allegra Strategies, entitled *Project Beauty – UK Salon and Spa Market*, was released in the UK in November 2003. This claimed that the current market comprises 12 370 outlets offering beauty treatments in the UK and is estimated to reach 14 425 by December 2005.

- Total revenue for salon-based outlets is forecasted to reach £1.15 billion by 2005 across 8855 units.
- Dynamic market growth is fuelled by consumers' desire to 'relax' and 'pamper' themselves.
- Increasingly busy lifestyles and a growing focus on personal well-being and appearance are driving visits to beauty salons and spas.
- Consumers increasingly view beauty treatments as 'essential' in modern UK lifestyles.
- Two-thirds of beauty salon customers visit salons more now than in the past, and nearly two-thirds visit for beauty and relaxation treatments at least once a month.
- Customers show strong loyalty to salons, less fidelity to product brands. 80 per cent of beauty salon customers are loyal to the salons they visit, while over half of customers 'often' or 'sometimes' change beauty product brands.

This study was based on interviews and analysis from industry leaders and what is claimed as the largest ever sample of beauty salon and spa customers. Areas covered in the report include market size and growth forecasts; charting the continued expansion of salon and spa outlets. The report also indicates customers' habits, preferences and trends as well as their perceptions of beauty products and services. This includes market trends, which are drivers of growth and future market evolution, as well as detailed profiles and analyses of the major branded salon and spa chains and key salon product and equipment suppliers.

The sources of information were 126 in-depth interviews with industry experts including salon and spa managers and beauty therapists, directors and marketing managers of major industry players, beauty product and equipment suppliers, major pharmacy chains and beauty retailers as well as industry associations.

926 consumer surveys in 28 cities and towns across the UK, including London, were conducted by the researchers.

In their summary the researchers claim that the UK beauty salon and spa industry is witnessing dynamic growth fuelled by increasing consumer demand.

The number of outlets offering beauty treatments is forecasted to grow 8 per cent each year from approximately 12 370 in 2003 to 14 425 in 2005. Total revenue for salon-based outlets is forecasted to grow at a rate of 11 per cent each year to reach £1.15 billion by 2005 across 8855 units.

The research indicates that beauty salons and spas are becoming more popular among UK consumers, who have increased their frequency of visits over the past 2–3 years. 66.1 per cent of the sample interviewed visit salons more frequently and 61.6 per cent visit salons for beauty and relaxation treatments at least once a month.

Driven by greater media coverage of beauty topics, increasingly busy lifestyles, and a growing focus on personal well-being and appearance, consumers of beauty salon and spas view beauty treatments as 'essential' in modern UK lifestyles. They visit salons not only to improve their appearance, but also to 'feel better', to 'pamper' themselves, and to have 'healthier skin'.

The main reasons for selecting a specific beauty salon or spa are convenience of location and the therapist at the salon. Strong personal relationships with individual therapists play an important role in fostering customer trust and loyalty, which is remarkably high: the research shows that 80 per cent of customers are loyal to the salon they visit.

However, 58 per cent of consumers surveyed change beauty product brands regularly ('often' or 'sometimes'). They like to experiment with new products – particularly when they perceive a decrease in the effectiveness of their current products, and when they receive product recommendations from therapists, friends and family.

The main considerations when purchasing beauty products are 'value for money,' products 'tailored to skin type,' and 'brand reputation. 61 per cent disagreed that higher prices relate to better quality.

Beauty products and services are appealing to a widening consumer base. The ageing UK population is driving growth in the demand for beauty, as are younger consumer groups for whom personal appearance is of increasing importance.

Spa's educational role

One aspect not covered by research is the spiritual. In the US survey 31 per cent of the respondents visited a spa to 'improve' their mental health. To be truly successful a spa has to have heart. Mel Zuckerman is one of the pioneers of the international spa industry and the founder of Canyon Ranch in Tucson, Arizona, which now has several branches, including The Venetian in Las Vegas and the spa on board the P&O cruise liner Queen Mary II. He received a letter from one of their first clients many years ago which read:

> *Thank you for taking my body to places it had never been and my spirit to places where it had always wanted to go.*

There can be few higher accolades than that!

Appendix A
i Spa Treatment Packages
ii Benefits of Spa Treatments
iii Spa Etiquette

Ai: SPA TREATMENT PACKAGES
3 HOUR SPA SEQUENCE

TREATMENT	DURATION
1. GREEK HERBAL BATH *A very mild sauna with low humidity and herbal aromatic steam*	15 MINUTES
2. EXPERIENCE SHOWER – 'Tropical' *Automatic aromatic shower with several options*	5 MINUTES
3. REFLEXOLOGY FOOTBATHS *A relaxing effervescent warm foot bath with heated individual seats*	10 MINUTES
4. LACONIUM *A relaxing dry aromatic room*	15 MINUTES
5. TURKISH HAMMAN *Roman style aromatic steam room*	10 MINUTES
6. EXPERIENCE SHOWER – 'Fresh' – cool minted mist *Automatic aromatic shower with several options*	5 MINUTES
7. MEDITATION ROOM – Rest Room *Rest room with heated ergonomic ceramic couches*	15 MINUTES
8. JAPANESE SALT BATH *Aromatic salt and steam atmosphere*	15 MINUTES
9. EXPERIENCE SHOWER – 'Rain' *Automatic aromatic shower with several options*	5 MINUTES
10. ZEN GARDEN *Outdoor Japanese garden of reflection*	5 MINUTES
11. TYROLEAN SAUNA *A Finnish dry heat treatment in a wood-lined room*	10 MINUTES
12. ICE ROOM *Cool room in which to rub crushed ice over the body*	5 MINUTES
13. SPA POOL *A warm pool with Hydro jets to massage the body*	15 MINUTES
14. EXPERIENCE SHOWER – 'Side or Splash' *Automatic aromatic shower with several options*	5 MINUTES
15. RELAX around the pool *Recommended to cool down and balance the body*	15 MINUTES
16. MASSAGE *A relaxing half hour massage*	30 MINUTES
TOTAL	180 MINUTES

It is recommended to drink several glasses of water in between each treatment to re-hydrate and detoxify the body

Ai: SPA TREATMENT PACKAGES – ZEN DAY
2 HOUR 45 MINUTES SPA SEQUENCE

TREATMENT	*DURATION*
1. JAPANESE SALT BATH *Aromatic salt and steam atmosphere*	20 MINUTES
2. EXPERIENCE SHOWER – 'Tropical' *Automatic aromatic shower with several options*	5 MINUTES
3. ZEN GARDEN *Outdoor Japanese garden of reflection*	5 MINUTES
4. REFLEXOLOGY BASINS *A relaxing effervescent warm foot-bath with heated individual seats*	10 MINUTES
5. EXPERIENCE SHOWER – 'Fresh' – cool minted mist *Automatic aromatic shower with several options*	5 MINUTES
6. MEDITATION ROOM – rest room *Rest room with heated ergonomic ceramic couches*	20 MINUTES
7. EXPERIENCE SHOWER – 'Rain' *Automatic aromatic shower with several options*	5 MINUTES
8. RELAX – with a refreshing cup of jasmine tea *Recommended to cool down and balance the body*	20 MINUTES
9. JAPANESE SILK BOOSTER FACIAL *Experience the ultimate in scientific skin therapy – Elemis*	75 MINUTES
TOTAL	165 MINUTES

It is recommended to drink several glasses of water in between each treatment to re-hydrate and detoxify the body

Ai: SPA TREATMENT PACKAGES – MOTHER TO BE
2 HOUR 30 MINUTES SPA SEQUENCE

TREATMENT	DURATION
1. EXPERIENCE SHOWER – 'Fresh' – cool minted mist *Automatic aromatic shower with several options*	5 MINUTES
2. REFLEXOLOGY BASINS *A relaxing effervescent warm footbath with heated individual seats*	10 MINUTES
3. MEDITATION ROOM – rest room *Rest room with heated ergonomic ceramic couches*	***20 MINUTES***
4. SPA POOL *A warm pool with Hydro jets to massage the body*	20 MINUTES
5. EXPERIENCE SHOWER – 'Tropical' *Automatic aromatic shower with several options*	5 MINUTES
6. ZEN GARDEN *Outdoor Japanese garden of reflection*	10 MINUTES
7. RELAX around the pool *Recommended to cool down and balance the body*	30 MINUTES
8. ELEMIS PREGNANCY CARE *A time to celebrate the wonders of nature*	50 MINUTES
	TOTAL 150 MINUTES

It is recommended to drink several glasses of water in between each treatment to re-hydrate and detoxify the body

Ai: SPA TREATMENT PACKAGES – THE EXOTIC SPA EXPERIENCE

3.10 HOUR SPA SEQUENCE

TREATMENT	DURATION
1. INDIAN BLOSSOM STEAM ROOM *An exotic aromatic warm and relaxing atmosphere*	15 MINUTES
2. EXPERIENCE SHOWER – 'Tropical' *Automatic aromatic shower with several options*	5 MINUTES
3. REFLEXOLOGY FOOTBATHS *A relaxing effervescent warm footbath with heated individual seats*	10 MINUTES
4. GREEK HERBAL BATH *A very mild sauna with low humidity and herbal aromatic steam*	15 MINUTES
5. EXPERIENCE SHOWER – 'Splash' *Automatic aromatic shower with several options*	5 MINUTES
6. TURKISH HAMMAN *Roman style aromatic steam room*	10 MINUTES
7. EXPERIENCE SHOWER – 'Fresh' – cool minted mist *Automatic aromatic shower with several options*	5 MINUTES
8. JAPANESE SALT BATH *Aromatic salt and steam atmosphere*	15 MINUTES
9. ICE FOUNTAIN *Cool room in which to rub crushed ice over the body*	5 MINUTES
10. ZEN GARDEN *Outdoor Japanese garden of reflection*	10 MINUTES
11. EXPERIENCE SHOWER – 'Side or Splash' *Automatic aromatic shower with several options*	5 MINUTES
12. AQUA MEDITATION ROOM *Recommended to cool down and balance the body*	15 MINUTES
13. CLEOPATRA SLIPPER POOL *A relaxing half hour massage*	30 MINUTES
14. DRY FLOAT *Cleopatra's milk bath wrap*	30 MINUTES
15. BODY SOFT *Application of Elemis Exotic body balm*	15 MINUTES
TOTAL	190 MINUTES

It is recommended to drink several glasses of water in between each treatment to re-hydrate and detoxify the body

www.spa-therapy.com   ©HCB Associates – Oct 2001

Aii: BENEFITS OF SPA TREATMENTS – AT A GLANCE

Serail

A relaxing therapeutic cleansing ceremony, using therapeutic muds, in a gentle herbal steam environment to exfoliate dead skin cells, eliminate toxins, increase circulation and leave the skin soft. Enhanced by light and sound effects to stimulate the five senses. *Temperature* operates between 35–45°C. *Duration* ½ hour.

Greek herbal bath

A very mild sauna with low humidity, with fresh herbal aromatic steam (camomile, sage and rosemary). Provides a gentle, warm, scented, mountain herb atmosphere. Relaxing and soporific, suitable for everyone as the preface to the complete spa experience. *Temperature* operates at 60°C and 60 per cent humidity. *Duration* 20 minutes.

Turkish hamman

Based upon a Roman-style steam room with an aromatic moist atmosphere (Eucalyptus) to either relax or stimulate the client, with light and sound effects to stimulate the five senses. The body heats up to stimulate the blood circulation initiating the purifying and detoxifying process. *Temperature* operates between 60–80°C, ambient air temperature with steam. *Duration* 10 minutes/shower/back in for 10 minutes.

Reflexology footbaths

A relaxing effervescent warm foot bath, stimulating the reflex zones of the feet, with heated seats. This provides a central area for interaction between spa goers and the experiences of the herb bath, laconium, sauna and ice room. *Temperature* operates between 38–45°C. *Duration* 5 minutes.

Laconium

A relaxing dry aromatic environment (orange), creating a Roman sauna atmosphere. The body gently heats up to stimulate the blood circulation initiating the purifying and detoxifying processes. *Temperature* operates between 45–60°C, with 15–20 per cent humidity. *Duration* 20–30 minutes.

Ice fountain

A contrast to a heat treatment such the Tyrolean sauna. Crushed ice, rubbed over the body, stimulates the circulation, lymphatic and immune system. Is used in medical spas to treat anxiety, stress and depression. *Temperature* operates at 15°C or less.

Tyrolean sauna

A Finnish dry heat treatment in a wood-lined room. The heat induces sweating to cleanse the body of impurities. The body gently heating up to stimulate the blood circulation, which initiates the purifying and detoxifying process. *Temperature* operates at 80–100°C. *Duration* 10 minutes/shower or ice/back in for 10 minutes.

Experience showers

The experience shower has several options:

1. **Fresh** – cold fog mist combined with a mint essence to enhance a feeling of coolness after a heat treatment
2. **Tropical** – rain-like massage shower using passion fruit essence invigorates you prior to a heat treatment
3. **Splash** – cold film of water from 4 jets – invigorating
4. **Rain** – cold
5. **Side** – 4 jets – warm
6. **Head** – cold.

Temperature – variable.

Relaxation/meditation room – tepidarium

This room consists of a relaxation area and heated ceramic ergonomic beds. You can stay in this room for long periods to relax. The heated ceramic ergonomic beds warm up your body which is ideal prior to massage treatments or also (or between) the other heat experiences. *Temperature* operates between 42–45°C. *Duration* 20–30 minutes.

Cleopatra slipper pool

This pool is a relaxing hydro-jet bath in a sensory haven of sound and light and aromatics to create an Egyptian experience. The Cleopatra slipper pool promotes relaxation as it soothes away aches and pains, releasing tension and stress as well as hydrating the skin. *Temperature* operates at 36°C. *Duration* 20 minutes.

Aqua meditation room

A relaxing, dry and warm aromatic environment with light and sound to stimulate the five senses. The guest relaxes on a cushioned reclining bench looking up at the light-reflected ripples of water on the ceiling whilst listening to calming music. Relax, reflect and contemplate. *Temperature* operates at 28°C. *Duration* 20–30 minutes.

Indian blossom steam room

An Indian-style steam room with an exotic aromatic atmosphere. Music, soft light and warmth stimulate the five senses, releasing tension and stress. *Temperature* operates between 42–45°C. *Duration* 20 minutes.

Japanese salt bath

A rose quartz crystal sits in the centre of the room with an automatic salt and aromatic (jasmine and mint) spray system. Humidity, essential oils and salt create an artificial sea atmosphere that opens the sinuses and clears the air passages. With heated seats and centre footrests. It is recommended that this is followed with a shower immediately after using the Japanese salt bath, before using any of the other spa experiences, to remove the salt from the skin, which could be drying. *Temperature* operates between 45–48°C, humidity 60 per cent, ambient air temperature. *Duration* 20 minutes.

Spa pool

The hydro-jets promote relaxation as it soothes away minor aches and pains, releasing tension and stress. The client feels healthier, invigorated and more energetic. *Temperature* operates at 30°C. *Duration* 20 minutes.

Dry Float

A complete and virtually instant relaxation treatment, where the body is cocooned in a waterproof sheet and literally dry floating, suspended in warm water, enveloped in a combination of aromatic products. *Temperature* operates at between 34–38°C. *Duration* 20 minutes.

Aiii: SPA ETIQUETTE

Questions answered to enable your guest to receive the maximum enjoyment from their visit to the spa

- **Should I reserve my treatments?**
- Yes, either by phone or visit the spa to book a reservation at your earliest convenience so that the spa can accommodate your schedule.

- **What should I wear?**
- Wear whatever is comfortable. The spa will provide you with a robe, slippers and a locker for your personal belongings.

- **When should I arrive?**
- Arrive at least 30 minutes prior to your treatment to relax and enjoy the luxurious facilities and amenities.

- **What do I wear during my treatment?**
- Most body treatments are enjoyed without clothing and the therapist will ensure you are modestly covered at all times.

- **Who can help me choose my treatments?**
- The spa receptionists will help you plan the perfect spa experience, including the best order in which to receive the treatments. Spa packages are designed to offer you a selection of the treatments available.

- **Where do I change my clothes?**
- In the spa locker and cloakroom, or arrive in your robe from your hotel room.

- **Should men shave before a facial?**
- Shaving isn't necessary but it is recommended. If you choose to shave prior to your facial then be sure to do so at least 2 hours prior to your scheduled appointment.

- **What if I have a special health consideration?**
- You will be asked to complete a medical questionnaire prior to your treatment.

- **What if I am late for my appointment?**
- Arriving late will simply limit the time for your treatment, thus lessening the effectiveness and your pleasure.

- **What if I need to cancel a spa treatment?**
An example of a Cancellation policy:
- Guests who do not cancel 4 hours in advance of the scheduled treatment will be charged 100 per cent of the fee.

- **Is there a pressure to talk during a treatment?**
- It is entirely the guest's choice. If you wish to be silent then the therapist will respect that. If you wish to ask a question throughout the treatment that is your prerogative.

- **What if I have a particular injury or physical condition?**
- The staff and therapists are trained to advise upon suitable treatments.

- **Can I choose to have a male or female therapist?**
- You will be asked your preferences at the time of booking a treatment.

- **What are the policies on tipping?**
- It's best to ask about the company's policy on tipping at the reception desk.

- **What is a spa 'Menu'?**
- This is a description of the treatment and its benefits, duration and cost of treatment.

- **What if a therapist's touch is too rough or too light?**
- You should explain this to your therapist – it is important to your therapist that you receive the perfect spa experience.

Appendix B
Spa education

Training courses in spa therapy are relatively new and, with the explosive growth of the spa business over the last 10 years now providing career opportunities in this sector, courses are now becoming abundant, some of which are of questionable value.

> *The Spa industry is a labour intensive service industry dependent upon the availability of good staff for its survival and its ability to deliver good quality services and products. The quality and availability of skilled staff is one of the major problems for the industry, which may be rectified through education and where possible, accurate careers information and guidance*

(Sarah Rawlinson, Curriculum Development and Quality Manager, The University of Derby, UK)

Table B.2 is a list of dedicated spa and leisure management courses.

The University of Derby

BSc. (Hons) international spa management

Stage one

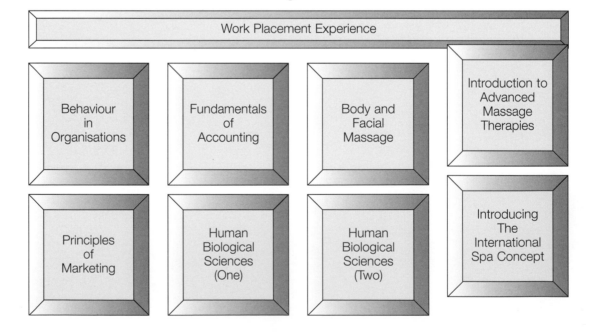

During stage one of the programme, students will begin to broaden their horizons by reading, comparing and contrasting information generated by management, therapy and spa experts. This process is underpinned by a module entitled 'Professional Studies and Information Technology'.

Through this module, students will begin to develop their research and presentation skills.

Three management modules introduce students to the concept of managing people, products and finance within the international spa environment.

The practical elements of the programme are supported by the study of 'Human Biological Sciences'. All students will be required to perform massage within a realistic working environment, thereby gaining first-hand experience of customer service, spatial and time considerations, essential to the smooth running of any therapy-based organisations.

Basic legislation, health and safety and customer scheduling are encountered through the module 'Introducing the International Spa Concept'.

Stage two

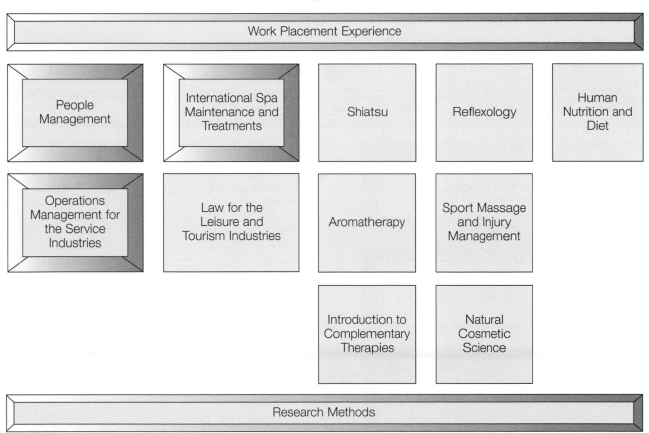

During stage two of the programme, students are required to attend a short work placement of 240 hours. This module is designed to enable students to synthesise their academic management and practical experiences from stage one into the working environment and to evaluate their own development by the application of transferable skills within the organisation.

Two management modules complete the suite of standard management experiences. However, students can opt to take a third management module entitled 'Law for the Leisure and Tourism Industries' if they wish to.

'International Spa Maintenance and Treatments' is a compulsory module that looks at the extensive range of international spa treatments within a practical setting, underpinned by a sound knowledge of health and safety issues, water chemistry and physics.

A suite of practical complementary and science based option modules are available to enhance student understanding of the therapy environment, not necessarily to develop students as practitioners but to integrate management considerations with practical skill acquisition. Students will be able to choose two option modules during this stage.

Stage three

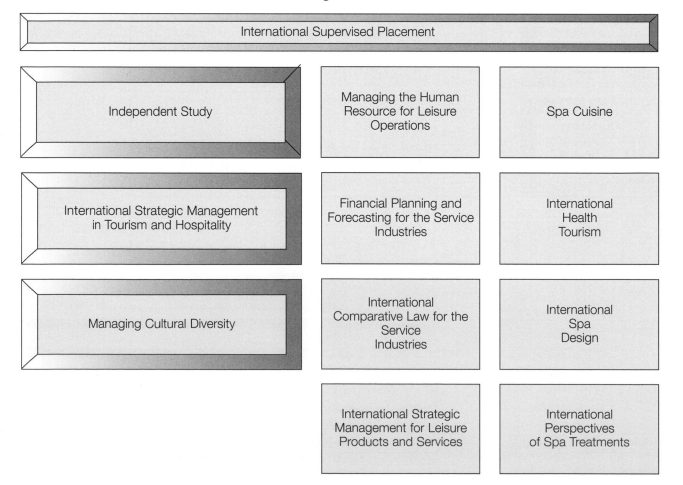

Finally, in preparation for stage three of the programme, students will study 'Research Methods'. Through this module, students will encounter paradigms, statistics and methods of presenting research data in preparation for their own research project.

Prior to stage three of the programme, students take a year out in the industry to consolidate their learning and prepare for more detailed and analytical research. The ability to apply concepts and become immersed in the industry will enhance and enrich the student learning experience at stage three.

During stage three of the programme, students will study three compulsory modules. 'Independent Study' which culminates in the production of a dissertation, 'International Strategic Management in Tourism and Hospitality' which draws on theoretical models specifically adapted and contextualised for these industries and 'Managing Cultural Diversity' which considers the difficulties of managing an international work force and an international clientele.

Students can then choose four option modules to conclude their programme. Of the eight options available, four are management based and four take an overview of the operational issues of international spa management. Students can opt to take a mixture of these two pathways.

HCB Associates spa seminars

HCB Associates conduct training seminars for those working or interested in the spa industry. These four days give an overview of the international spa industry. They are designed to be interactive, and can be adapted to the needs of the participants.

HCB Associates deliver these workshops in the UK, Europe, Asia Pacific, South Africa and Australia.

Learning outcome of day one:

Day one will enable students to have a good understanding of the background to global spa culture, and an introduction to global spa therapies and their benefits.

To include:

- *Physical properties of water*
- *Physiological changes during immersion in water*
- *Treating the five senses*
- *Spa treatments and procedures*

One day	One day	Two days
History of spa – Time line	Spa criteria – the ten elements	Research, surveys and market trends – including general marketing of spas and wellness
Global spa developments	Spa maintenance	Review of manufactured spa equipment
Global spa treatments		The future
Spa etiquette	Filtration, microbiology and water testing; water borne disease	Spa project analysis and design
Psychological and physiological effects of spa treatments	Strategies for managing a successful spa business	Design concepts
Product use	Marketing	Project viability and budgets
Exercise in spas Ai Chi	Total quality management	Project management
Spa experience/or Ai Chi session in spa pool	Service	Project recommendations
	Recruitment	Project development
	Leadership	Report writing

Table B.1 HCB Associates' spa seminal outline

- *Workshop – spa experience*
  - *– demonstration of Dry Float bed*
  - *– Ai Chi session in the pool*
  - *– treatment session*

Learning outcome of day two:

Day two will enable students to have a full understanding of the operational safety guidelines and strategic planning necessary for a successful spa business. This day will be a benefit to those moving into management roles within their company.

To include:

- *Marketing*
- *Service*
- *Recruitment*
- *Leadership*
- *Total quality management*
- *Report writing*

Learning outcome of day three:

Day three will enable students to have an understanding of the spa and wellness business and its market trends. This day looks at the role of 'spa consultant' and how to build an effective project team.

To include:

- *Appointing an effective design team*
- *Mechanical and electrical (M & E)*
- *Filtration and drainage*
- *Water choice*
- *Health and safety*
- *Operational do's and don'ts – stretching the design parameters*
- *Traffic flow*
- *Treatment rooms*
- *Plant rooms*

Learning outcome of day four:

Day four continues with the theme of spa design and gives the student an opportunity to analyse architectural plans and real life situations by considering the issues involved in designing a spa. This will enable students to have a good understanding of design concepts and constraints.

To include:

- *Project recommendations*
- *Budgets – realistic and achievable*
- *Project management*
- *Project development*
- *Design for safety – responsibilities and regulations*
- *Choosing competent contractors and subcontractors*

	MSA (Master of Spa Administration)	*CSP (Certified Spa Practitioner)*	*Seminar Spa Programme*	*Seminar Spa Experience*
Tuition goal	Spa manager qualified to set up and manage a spa	Spa practitioner qualified to for holistic care and overseeing spa programmes	Knowledge about holistic spa programmes	Experience of a holistic spa programme with background information
Duration/ structure	Part-time study 2 years 700 €E	Part-time study 2 years 700 €E	A 7-day week with spa experience	3-day experience with 2 hours' theory daily

www.spa-academy.de

	MSA (Master of Spa Administration)	CSP (Certified Spa Practitioner)	Seminar Spa Programme	Seminar Spa Experience
Tuition content	Management and marketing product programme planning; charge policy; communication/ event/facility/ finance/personnel development and quality management; health/prophylaxis naturopathy/TCM fitness/exercise/ beauty care/ dermatology/ physical therapy/ nutrition/dietetics communications/ psychology	Health/prophylaxis naturopathy/TCM fitness/exercise/ beauty care/ dermatology/ physical therapy/ nutrition/dietetics communications/ psychology; management/ marketing	Management/ marketing; naturopathy/TCM fitness/exercise/ beauty care/ dermatology/ physical therapy/ nutrition/dietetics; communications/ psychology/health/ prophylaxis	Naturopathy/TCM fitness/exercise/ beauty care/ dermatology/ physical therapy/ nutrition/ dietetics/health/ prophylaxis
Participants	Hotel managers, health resort mgrs, health resort physicians, fitness trainers	physiotherapists, fitness trainers, cosmeticians, hairdressers	Managers of hotels, health resorts, hotels, rehabilitation centres, spas and associated fields	Executive personnel from industry and administration, professional fitness instructors
Requirements	Degree, appropriate experience	Fully qualified in a relevant profession, professional experience, participation in a recognised course, related profession		
Fees	Complete course with MSA certificate €18,000; grant from sponsor company	Complete course with CSP certificate €10,000; grant from sponsor company	Seminar € 3,000; suitable as an incentive programme	Seminar € 2,000; suitable as an incentive programme

Table B.2 The European Spa Academy course programme

The Rogner Academy

'Rogner Spa Apprenticeship'

This comprises of modular training and seminar programmes in the field of spa and health tourism. Developing skills in social competency through personality training seminars, professional knowledge in spa and health tourism and standards that the discerning spa-goer now expects.

This modular qualification programme consists of two-day seminars held several times during the apprenticeship and includes:

- *Catering for health tourism*
- *Basic knowledge of holistic treatment methods*
- *Sports and leisure tourism*
- *Social skills and etiquette*
- *Communication*
- *TQM – total quality management*
- *Hands-on learning IT skills*

LIVING SYSTEMS❶ Professional Spa Training Series

The Spa Center, 121N Churton Street, Hillsborough, North Carolina 27278 USA.

www.thespacenter.com   Tel:+1 888 678 0882

Living Systems❶ offers courses approved by the National Certification Board for Therapeutic Massage and Bodywork (NCBTMB) as a continuing education provider under category A.

Sample of courses offered:

Eight-day intensive

The Eight Day Intensive consists of a combination of the five separate courses and costs (2002) $1,599

Skills covered:

Foundations in Spa Therapies

- *Foundations in spa philosophy and ethics*
- *Foundations in aromatherapy*
- *Introductions to spa reflexology*
- *Hot herbal resting wrap*
- *Aromatherapy wrap*
- *Localised body treatments*
- *Facial mask/massage techniques*

Giving the Waters 1[0]; Exfoliation and the Wet Room

- *Fundamentals of hydrotherapy*
- *Exfoliating procedures including body polishes and salt glows with and without hydro-kinetic Vichy or Swiss shower*
- *Wet room set-up and sanitation*

Giving the Waters 1[0]; Exfoliation and the Wet Room

- *Foundations in thalassotherapy and peliotherapy*
- *Full body wrapping technique with and without hydro-kinetic Vichy or Swiss shower*
- *Simple and effective add-on services with full body wrap*

The Art of Bathing

- *Foundations of balneotherapy*
- *Properties of thermalism*
- *Physiological effects of water*
- *Contra-indications*
- *Types/varieties of soaking baths*
- *Basics of underwater massage*

Owning and Developing your Day Spa

- *Feasibility and planning*
- *Financial guidelines*
- *Layout and room design*
- *Staffing and training*
- *Marketing and sales tips*

Reference: Robin Zill, President, The spa Center Inc, spa training and Ousia spa therapy program, Great Spa Conversation – columnist. Email: robin@thespacenter.com

The Institute of Sports and Recreation Management (ISRM)

Recognised in the UK by the Department for Education and Employment under the 1992 Further and Higher Education Act, the local authority associations, the Local Government Management Board, the Health and Safety Executive and Sports England.

The programme comprises modular learning over 2 years with day release at college. There are 4 levels of training.

Institute of Sport and Recreation Management

Gifford House, 36–38 Sherrard Street, Melton Mowbray, Leicestershire LE13 1XJ UK.

Tel: +44 (0)1664 565531.

International Spa and Aesthetics (ISA)

The educational division of Spa Synergy has linked up with the Tourism Management Institute of Singapore (www.tmis-edu.com) to create management based seminars. The programme includes:

- *Business policy and marketing*
- *Finance and operations*
- *Human resources*
- *Management communications*
- *Site visits to Spas*
- *Guest speakers from the industry*

Cost of programme: $1,980

International Spa Association (ISPA)

ISPA and the ISPA Foundation have partnered with the Educational Institute of the American Hotel and Lodging Association (EI) to deliver Supervisory Skill Builders certified programme and books for the spa industry. The books and certified programme can be found online at www.experienceispa.com

Glossary

accupressure   an ancient form of Chinese medicine using fingertip pressure on the meridian points of the body to channel energy

aerobics   exercise regime set to music to increase blood circulation and increase the aerobic capacity of the heart and lungs

affusion shower   relaxing shower of warm droplets of water – seawater, mineral or aromatic, whilst lying on a couch. A lymph drainage massage can also be given

Ai Chi   created using a combination of Eastern and Western methods of tai chi, shiatsu and aquatic exercise to stimulate both the mind and body

Alexander Technique   a massage system created to correct physical habits of posture that cause stress

algotherapy   the therapeutic use of algae or marine based products to detoxify, rebalance and relax the body

aqua aerobics   gentle gymnastics in the water, sometimes using water jets to increase resistance and tone up the muscles

aromatherapy   an ancient therapeutic practice of utilising essential oils from plants, leaves, bark, roots, seeds, resins and flowers used in pressure point massage, hydrotherapy, face and body treatments

Aslan therapy   developed in Romania, Gerovital H3 or Aslavital drug therapy using for their regenerative effect in fighting the ageing process

ayurveda   an ancient Eastern Indian philosophy and practice of traditional folk medicine using herbs, aromatherapy, nutrition, massage and meditation to create a balance between the mind and body

Bach flower cures   the use of flowers for healing

balneotherapy   water therapy treatments using mineral, sea or hot springs water to alleviate stresses and strains within the body

basti   Ayurvedic herbal purification treatment

bindi   body treatment combining exfoliation, herbal treatment and light massage

body composition analysis   a method used to determine the ratio of body fat to lean muscle

body scrub (exfoliation)   exfoliation of dead skin cells using various combinations of sea salt, essential oils, water, skin brush or loofah to massage the body and leave the skin silky soft

body sugaring   ancient practice of hair removal using sugar

breema bodywork   the practice of breema, from the mountains of Kurdistan, is designed to create harmony and balance the mind and body

brine baths   water that is saturated with salt (sodium chloride), similar to the sea

brossage   a fine body polish using salicylic salt and brushes

brush and tone   body exfoliating treatment using skin brushes, as a pre-envelopment treatment or followed by a hydrating oil or cream massage

caldarium   an aromatic steam room

cathiodermie   a rejuvenating skin treatment using galvanic and high frequency currents of electric stimulation in a low voltage dose to deep cleanse and improve circulation

Celtic Roman bath   a sequence of hot and cold baths, showers and pools combined with heat and steam rooms

chi   outward energy

chiropractic   the realignment of the spine and bone/body mechanics in order to relieve backache and postural problems

circuit training   exercise regime using a series of weight training devices combining the resistance with aerobics

climatotherapy   the physiological effects of the use of unique qualities of air and climate on the human body involving, temperature, atmospheric pressure, humidity, air purity, light, sun, wind and location

coenocytic   a mass of protoplasm that contains many nuclei and is enclosed by a cell wall

cold plunge   deep cold water pool to stimulate blood circulation and rapidly cool the body, especially after a sauna

colonic irrigation   water cleansing of the colon to help detoxify the body

Colour Therapy (colour analysis)   an analysis of colours to suit and complement your skin shades to determine whether you are a spring, summer, autumn or winter colour type

Colour Therapy (colour healing)   an ancient philosophy of the vibration of colour that attracts a similar vibration in the human body

cortisol   also known as hydrocortisone, is an important glucocorticoid produced by the adrenal gland on top of the kidney

cranio-sacral therapy   a gentle massage that centres on the head and neck

crenotherapy   any treatment incorporating mineral water, mud and vapour

cross training   alternating high and low stress exercises or sports to enhance mental and physical conditioning

cryotherapy   the use of very cold or frozen products to vaso-constrict the skin and muscle and create a lift in the skin

crystal healing   the use of crystals to draw out an imbalanced energy from the body

cymatics   pioneered by British osteopath, Sir Peter Manners in the 1960's – cymatics is sound therapy, also known as bioresonance or vibrational therapy. He developed a machine using a healing vibrations system, set at a certain frequency, to match the cells of a healthy body, encouraging the body's cells to vibrate at a healthy resonance

dancercise   aerobic exercise routine derived from modern dance

Dead Sea mud therapy   applications of a mineral rich mud from the Dead Sea to detoxify the skin and body

deep (tissue) muscle massage   a deep muscle massage to help realign the body and give freedom of movement

doshas   Ayurvedic body functions: vata for blood, circulation and healing, pitta for heat and metabolism, and kapha for the structure of one's spiritual and philosophical self

douche à jet   *see* Scottish douche

dulse scrub   exfoliating body scrub with a mixture of dulse seaweed powder, oil and water to deep cleanse and re-mineralise the skin. Leaves the skin incredibly smooth

duo massage   synchronous massage by two therapists

endermologie   a French massage therapy that reduces the appearance of cellulite

Esalen massage   a massage that combines Swedish and sensory relaxation techniques to harmonise the whole body

esters   compounds produced by a reaction between acids and alcohol when the water has been removed. Esters are responsible for the fragrance of a plant

exfoliation   the removal of dead skin cells using products, loofah rub or body brush

fango therapy   highly mineralised mud, rich in nutrients to deep cleanse, purify and revitalise the skin

flexercise   stretching and toning exercises to increase flexibility

flotation tank   the combination of a darkened room and a shallow pool of salt or Epsom salts to enable the body to float, inducing deep relaxation

free radicals   molecules with an unpaired electron that are therefore unstable

golden needles   an anti-wrinkle facial program at Clinic La Prairie. The insertion of golden needles to stimulate blood circulation and strengthen relaxed muscles

golden spoons   alternating hot and cold 23 carat gold-plated spoons on the face to stimulate circulation and help the absorption of creams and lotions

hamman   Turkish or Middle Eastern communal bath house

haysack wrap   Kneipp treatment using steamed organic Alpine hay to detoxify the body

Hellerwork   Joseph Heller devised a programme of eleven 90-minute sessions of deep tissue bodywork and movement to realign the body and release chronic tension and stress

herbal wrap   the body is wrapped in herb-soaked hot linen sheets and then covered in blankets, a cool compress is applied to the forehead. Herbal wraps help relax the muscles, detoxify and soften the skin

hot mineral spring   a natural, sometimes volcanic, spring of hot mineral water

hot tub   a wooden tub of hot or cool water to soak the body

hydro massage   an underwater massage in a hydro bath equipped with high pressure jets and hand-manipulated hose

hydro pool   a pool equipped with various high pressure jets, air beds and neck fountains

hydrostatic pressure   the sideways pressure applied to an immersed body

hydrotherapy   term meaning any therapeutic use of water

infrared treatment   a heat treatment to aid muscular relaxation

inhalation therapy   treatments involving the inhalation of steam vapour combined with essential oils

Japanese enzyme bath   relaxing and detoxifying treatment in a wooden tub filled with fragrant blends of cedar fibres and Japanese plant enzymes, which stimulate the circulation. You are served a refreshing hot enzyme tea

Japanese facial energising technique, to stimulate the acupressure points on the face and scalp

Jet Blitz *see* Scottish douche

jinn shin jyutsu a form of energy balancing massage

jin shin do a form of energy balancing massage

Jungian therapy therapy based on the work of Carl G. Jung that focuses on the realisation of personality by exploring the subconscious

kinesiology diagnosis and treatment of a disease through muscle testing

kirlian photography a special photographic technique that shows the energy field surrounding the body

Kneipp baths herbal/mineral baths of varying temperatures combined with diet and exercise

Kneipp Kur System the five pillars of Kneipp – hydro, phyto, kinesi, dietetic and regulative. Treatments combining hydrotherapy, herbology and a diet of natural foods developed by Father Sebastian Kneipp to achieve physical and emotional well- being

laconium an evenly distributed dry heat treatment room

lap pool a shallow swimming pool with exercise lanes

liquid balancing floating in salt water at body temperature

Liquid Sound light and music under and above water for relaxation and visualisation

loofah body scrub dried plant used as a friction massage to exfoliate the body

lomi lomi Hawaiian rhythmical, rocking massage

lymphatic drainage massage a therapeutic massage using a gentle pumping technique to reduce pockets of water retention. Lymph drainage can be achieved through manual, hydro or aromatherapy massage

marine hydrotherapy a form of thalassotherapy bath/shower, where water jets massage the body

mandala a mandala consists of a series of concentric forms, suggestive of a passage between different dimensions

mariel a form of energy balancing massage

meditation a form of focusing on a specific thought, memory and breathing which encourages the body to relax and achieve a greater sense of inner balance and peace

mineral water bath soaking in hot or cold mineral spring water

Moor peat baths a natural peat rich in organic matter used to ease pains and stiffness

morphology specialised form of massage with essential oils that targets the digestive areas

naturopathy   the discipline of natural medicine and healing through the power of nature and all natural substances

NIA   non-impact aerobics – not as rigorous as traditional aerobic exercise

nuat Thai   a form of energy balancing massage

nutrition counselling   consultation with a qualified nutritional practitioner to review an individual's eating habits and dietary needs

oedema   retention of fluid in the body causing swelling

oleation   Ayurvedic adapted friction massage treatment using blended essential oils

onsen   a Japanese natural mineral thermal spring

oxygen facials   oxygen and other nutrients applied to the face to stimulate and reinforce the collagen level of the skin

ozonised baths   a tub of thermal water or seawater with a system of jets that provide streams of ozonised bubbles, used for relaxation and stimulation of circulation

panchakarma   Ayurvedic cleansing and purification treatment using essential oils, massage and meditation

parafango   combination of fango mud and paraffin wax to detoxify, heat and exfoliate

parcours   outdoor exercise trail with exercise stations along the way provided with instructions and equipment for various exercises and obstacles designed to be fun and challenging

pelotherapy   treatments utilising mud or mud products

physiochineitherapy   therapeutic use of light, heat, electrical and mechanical means to regenerate strength and flexibility

phytotherapy   healing treatment through plants, herbs, aromatic essential oils and seaweeds applied through massage, wraps, steam therapies, inhalation and herbal teas

Pilates   exercise routine of stretching and strengthening the body through coordinated breathing techniques

polarity massage   a technique of gently rocking, holding and massaging the body, designed to balance the body's subtle or electromagnetic energy through touch, stretching exercises, diet and mental–emotional balanced attitude

qi   innermost energy

radon therapy   an inert gas used in many European spas as part of a treatment process to stimulate organ functions

Rasul bath   a cleansing ceremony using different grades of mud from fine for delicate areas of the body to deep cleansing coarser muds that are baked on the body whilst sitting on ceramic seats underneath a planetarium ceiling. A tropical rain shower of warm droplets of water washes the mud away and the treatment is finished with an application of oil

re-birthing   an extension of yogic breathing technique combined with guided meditation that allows total relaxation and clearing of the mind

reflexology   Ancient Egyptian, Chinese and Indian technique using finger point pressure on the reflex zones of the feet and hands to restore the flow of energy through the body

regression therapy   healing through being taken back to previous states or past experiences

Reiki   a technique of channeling energy to balance the body

rolfing   a technique of deep muscular manipulation and massage for the relief of rigid muscles, bones and joints, to relieve stress and emotional trauma

Roman bath –(see Celtic Roman bath)   ancient cleansing sequence of varying water temperatures, heated rooms, mineral pools and relaxation

Rubenfield synergy method   a practice developed by Llana Rubenfeld of merging body and mind through verbal expression and gentle touch

salt glow   a hydrating and exfoliating treatment consisting of salt, essential oils and water

sauna   a Finnish dry heat treatment in a wood-lined room, the heat induces sweating to cleanse the body of impurities

Scottish douche   standing body massage delivered by a therapist with a high pressure hose of alternating warm and cold water to stimulate the circulation and relieve tension

seaweed wrap   an envelopment of warm seaweed on the body, wrapped in a heated blanket to remineralise, revitalise and rebalance the body

shamanism   spiritual and natural healing performed by a medicine man

shiatsu   Japanese finger pressure technique, working the energy meridians to stimulate the body's inner powers of balance and healing

shirodhara   Ayurvedic treatment of warmed oil slowly pouring over the third eye in the centre of the forehead to induce deep relaxation

siddha vaidya   Ayurvedic massage treatment using a pouch of blended herbs dipped in essential oils and massage over the body

siliceous thermal bath – hot sand   treatment using silica

sitz bath   a chair-like bath where the hips and lower body are immersed in herbal hot water while the feet are soaking in alternating hot and cold water to stimulate the immune system

Slenisuim body wrap   a detoxifying body envelopment treatment using natural oils to stimulate the immune system

spinning   an aerobic form of exercise class using special stationary bicycles

sports massage   deep tissue massage on muscles used in athletic activities

steam room   an area of wet hot steam, that softens and cleanses the skin and relaxes the body

sweat lodge   an ancient Native American body purification ceremony using intense heat, similar to a sauna to stimulate vision and insight

Swedish massage   massage technique using firm but gentle pressure

tai chi (chuan)   a Chinese Taoist martial art discipline of meditation in movement using slow, controlled deep breathing techniques together with slow graceful physical movements

terpenes   are from a group of unsaturated hydrocarbons that are found in the essential oils of plants, in particular, conifers and citrus. Terpenes are obtained by distillation or extraction

Thai herbal heat treatment   a traditional herbal massage using Pai root, tamarind leaves and essentail oils to relax tired muscles

thalassotherapy   therapeutic use of seawater and marine by-products that are rich in minerals and vitamins to restore the balance of the body

thallus   from the Greek meaning 'green shoot', is the undifferentiated part of the body of algae

thermo-auricular therapy   the use of herbal Hopi Indian ear candles to cleanse the ear

Tomatis   sound therapy, also known as 'listening therapy' was developed by Dr Alfred Tomatis a French ear, nose and throat specialist, in the early 1950's. It is used to treat learning disabilities, behavioural problems, and depression to anxiety for children and adults. It also helps with co-ordination and motor problems. Tomatis involves the use of specially made headphones using bone and air conduction to listen to electronically recorded music frequencies. There are 250 Tomatis centres around the world (as at June 2000)

tonicité   bracing effect

Traeger massage   a gentle rhythmic shaking or rocking of the body to release tension from the joints that was developed by hawaiian physician Dr Milton Traeger

Turkish hamman bath   *see* hamman bath

ultra sound   high frequency sound waves to alleviate pain and discomfort to injured parts of the body

Vichy shower (affusion shower)   multi-jet shower of
  varying temperatures and pressures, which are often
  infused with aromatics suspended over a wet table –
  very relaxing

vision quest   Native American tradition and old native
  culture's rite of passage. A call for a period of time to be
  alone with nature

visualisation   a form of light hypnosis used to create a
  soothing environment for relaxation

Watsu   a method of rhythmic movements, pressure point
  massage and stretching the body, working with a
  therapist, in warm water that leads to state of deep
  relaxation

Wheel of Sri   known as sri yantra; yantras originate from
  religions such as Buddhism or Hinduism, and are
  geometric shapes intended to focus the mind in
  meditation

whirlpool   a heated pool with high pressure jets that
  circulate the water and relax the body

yoga   an ancient Hindu discipline composed of focused
  deep breathing, stretching and toning the body using
  various positions designed to improve circulation,
  flexibility and strength. A philosophical approach to
  balancing the body and mind

Zen   stresses the personal experience of enlightenment
  based on a simple life lived close to nature, and upon
  methods of meditation which avoid complicated rituals
  and abstruse thought.

Index

Note: Page numbers in *italics* refer to illustrations.